THE
Essential
Arthritis
Cookbook

Kitchen Basics for People with Arthritis, Fibromyalgia and Other Chronic Pain and Fatigue

Authored by the Arthritis Center
and the Department of Nutrition Sciences,
University of Alabama at Birmingham

First Edition

APPLETREE PRESS, INC.

Mankato, Minnesota

Appletree Press, Inc.
151 Good Counsel Drive, Suite 125
Mankato, MN 56001
Phone: (507) 345-4848
Fax: (507) 345-3002
Website: http://www.appletree-press.com

Cataloging-in-Publication Data
The Essential Arthritis Cookbook: Kitchen basics for people with arthritis, fibromyalgia, and other chronic pain and fatigue / authored by the Arthritis Center and the Department of Nutrition Sciences, University of Alabama at Birmingham; Sarah L. Morgan, et al. Birmingham, AL : University of Alabama, c1995, 1999, 2002.
    288 p. :ill., photos.; 23 cm.
    Includes indexes.
    Summary: The Essential Arthritis Cookbook is filled with information relating to arthritis and nutritional status. Important points covered by this book include: arthritis medications and their effect on diet, when arthritis and the medications taken make eating difficult, how to overcome kitchen energy robbers, adaptive equipment and tool catalog lists and the use of convenience foods to conserve energy. Over 120 original, low-fat recipes that save time and energy with nutrition analysis and diabetic exchanges provided.
    ISBN-10: 1-891011-01-4
    ISBN-13: 978-1-891011-01-6
    1. Arthritis—Nutritional aspects. 2. Arthritis—Diet therapy—Recipes. 3. Cookery for the sick. 4. Low-cholesterol Diet—Recipes. I. Title: Arthritis cookbook. II. University of Alabama. Department of Nutrition Sciences. III. University of Alabama. Arthritis Center. IV. Morgan, Sarah L.
RM221   99-64650
641.563

First-Fifth printing: 102,000 copies

Editors: Linda Hachfeld and Faith Winchester
Assistant: Johnna Solting
Cover Design: Douglas Allan Graphic Design

Printed in the United States of America

CONTRIBUTORS

Sarah L. Morgan M.D., M.S., R.D., F.A.C.P.
Janet S. Austin M.Ed., Ph.D.
Lisa L. Hughes M.S., R.D.
Nedra P. Wilson M.S., R.D.
Annie R. Cornwell M.S., R.D.
Louise R. Thibodaux M.A., O.T.R., F.A.O.T.A.
Carol B. Craig M.S., R.D.

Departments of Nutrition Sciences, Applied Health Sciences,
Internal Medicine (Division of Clinical Immunology and Rheumatology),
Schools of Health Related Professions and Medicine,
The University of Alabama at Birmingham

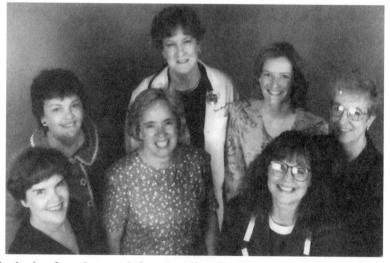

Clockwise from bottom left and ending in center: Annie Cornwell, Carol Craig, Sarah Morgan (in white coat), Lisa Hughes, Nedra Wilson, Janet Austin, Louise Thibodaux

The UAB Research Foundation gratefully acknowledges
the assistance of the following people in the preparation of this book:

Barbara Barnard, R.D.
Rebecca Bradley, MA., R.D.
Kathy Franklin
Virginia Hughes
Lisa Freeman, M.S., R.D.
Sarah McCleskey, Artist
Debra Richardson
Jerry Snead
Myra Thompson
Pearl Williamson, D.T.R.

A special thanks to the Focus Group Participants:

Virginia Allen
Donald Bearden
Loretta Berube
Thelma Borter
Elvada Brickell
Faye P. Brown
Winifred Bryant
Billie Buchanan
Sara Coe
Marjorie S. Cooke
Mary Crow
Ollie M. Dixon
Sharon Dorough
Mary Jo Essix
Margo Fallin

Earline Fowler
Lillian Freed
Rema Friedman
Mira Griffith
Marguerite Hancock
Marion Helsley
Martha H. Hood
Bertha Johnson
Roberta Jones
Gladys Mitchell
Helen Montgomery
Wyllodene Mulkey
Joni Odess
Myra Odess
Beverly Parrish

Martha Ray
Edith A. Russell
Virginia Siniard
Josie Spruill
Geneva M. Taylor
Lenore Unger
Louise Williamson

Acknowledgements:
National Institutes of Health
Department of Research Resources Clinical Research Center: Grant RR-32-31S1
USPHS: Grants 5P01-CA-28103 and 5P60-AR-20614.

THE ESSENTIAL ARTHRITIS COOKBOOK
is highly recommended!

While nutrition therapy does not now have a consistent or established role in the management of most forms of arthritis, it is important that arthritis sufferers prepare food adequately and eat properly. **The Essential Arthritis Cookbook,** *whose senior author is both a physician and registered dietitian, will help patients achieve this. It presents thoughtful, balanced and useful information that will be valuable.*

Richard S. Panush, MD, Professor and Chairman
Department of Medicine
St. Barnabus Medical Center
UMDNJ—New Jersey Medical School

The Essential Arthritis Cookbook *is an invaluable resource for anyone with sensitive hands or upper extremity problems. It provides all the information necessary to prepare nutritious meals with limited energy and preparation time. It also gives accurate information on how diet impacts arthritis, which is difficult to find in most materials and books.*

Jenny Fransen, RN, Director, Arthritis Care Program
Abbott Northwestern Hospital, Minneapolis

Practical, no nonsense, savvy advice from real experts which cuts through much of the confusion about diet and arthritis.

Joel M. Kremer, MD, Professor of Medicine
Head, Division of Rheumatology, Albany Medical College

Much more than a cookbook, **The Essential Arthritis Cookbook** *attacks potential problems from every angle . . . And of the 123 down-to-earth recipes, 40 are tagged* **Quick & Easy***. In addition, there are sections on nutritional strategies that improve some types of arthritis; fatigue-fighting tips on arranging your kitchen; cooking tools that are easy on the joints; basic medication information . . . and more.*

Arthritis Newsletter, Remedy Magazine

After 13 years of living with arthritis, this book finally clears up some of the confusion about how my diet can affect my arthritis. It also addresses how my medications affect my diet which most books overlook.

Bonnie Raymond, RN, MS, Volunteer & Board Member
Arthritis Foundation-Minnesota Chapter

The Essential Arthritis Cookbook is an excellent resource for people with arthritis and other chronic illnesses. It includes a balanced presentation of the current state of knowledge about diet and arthritis, as well as an excellent selection of low-fat, easy to make recipes. The inclusion in the recipes of rest breaks and work tips to help protect joints is a terrific feature!

Ronenn Roubenoff, MD, MHS, FACP
Assistant Professor of Medicine and Nutrition, Tufts University
Rheumatologist, New England Medical Center

The Essential Arthritis Cookbook dispels many misconceptions surrounding arthritis and nutrition while providing so much practical information to help people with arthritis, like myself, minimize chronic pain and fatigue while working in the kitchen.

Janet Austin, PhD, Director
Arthritis Information Services—UAB

The Essential Arthritis Cookbook is an important resource for anyone who wants to feel well and who is interested in good health through nutrition.

Roland L. Weinsier, MD, DrPH, Professor and Chairman
Department of Nutrition Sciences, Univ. of Alabama at Birmingham

The Essential Arthritis Cookbook takes your special needs into account—the recipes are easy to prepare; there are few ingredients, and there is minimal clean-up. Adaptive equipment, kitchen lay-out, time-saving and special meal preparation methods are suggested.

Sarah L. Morgan, MD, RD, FACP, Principal Author
Associate Professor of Medicine, Department of Nutrition Sciences
Univ. of Alabama at Birmingham

The recipes and nutritional advice offered in The Essential Arthritis Cookbook will be extremely helpful to those with arthritis. It is clear that a well-balanced, sensible nutritional program is an important factor in the well-being of all of us.

William J. Koopman, MD,
Director, UAB Multipurpose and Musculoskeletal Diseases Center
Univ. of Alabama at Birmingham

Also. . .

This book has been reviewed by the Arthritis Foundation, which particularly likes the following elements:

Manageability of ingredients, utensils and time
Nutrition analysis on every recipe
Tips and rationales for people with arthritis

Table of Contents

Tables and Other Illustrations

Foreword

One of the most frequent concerns raised in the clinic by patients with arthritis relates to the relationship between diet and their arthritis. In this book, the authors discuss several aspects of this topic. As they point out, generally we have little evidence that foods, per se, trigger or exacerbate arthritis. A well known exception is gout, "the arthritis of royalty," which clearly can be exacerbated by dietary excesses (food and drink).

An active area of current research relates to the influence of dietary constituents on the body's immune defense system. These studies are in their infancy but have provided strong evidence that the nature of the dietary fats we eat can influence several aspects of the inflammatory response which contributes to tissue damage in several forms of arthritis. The role of certain vitamins in regulating inflammatory and immune processes in the body is being studied at several centers. These studies have indicated that vitamin A, for example, can diminish inflammation in several experimental systems. Investigators are interested in the role of folic acid, a common vitamin, in regulating the immune system. This interest has been prompted by promising experience with the antifolate compound methotrexate in the treatment of rheumatoid arthritis.

Better understanding of the precise mechanisms underlying the effectiveness of this antifolate may lead to the development of more effective, less toxic agents for the treatment of chronic inflammatory diseases. Nutritional research offers promise of providing new insights concerning the relationship between diet and arthritis. The recipes and nutritional advice offered in THE ESSENTIAL ARTHRITIS COOKBOOK will be extremely helpful to patients with arthritis. It is clear that a well-balanced, sensible nutritional program is an important factor in the well-being of all of us.

William J. Koopman, M.D.
Howard L. Holley Professor and Chairman of Medicine
Spencer Chair in Medicine Science Leadership
Director, UAB Multipurpose Arthritis and Musculoskeletal Diseases Ctr.
University of Alabama at Birmingham

Preface

A recent medical study demonstrated that careful attention to a healthy diet can result in significant improvement in the pain, swelling, and stiffness that accompanies arthritis. This is, not wholly new information, but it is an important confirmation that what we eat may impact directly on our well-being, especially if we suffer from arthritis. That is not to say that everyone and every type of arthritis will benefit equally. However, it means that there is good reason to take care of ourselves with the expectation that, in the long-term, healthier eating habits will translate to a healthier body.

Even in the short-term there are also ways to change your eating and cooking habits to begin feeling better: food preparation tips that make cooking easier for all of us, but especially when we have pain in our joints; shopping for convenience foods that are healthy and fit into a balanced diet; and even making some rearrangements in our kitchen to make the whole process of meal preparation easier. These are examples of how THE ESSENTIAL ARTHRITIS COOKBOOK addresses the needs of people with arthritis, as well as those of us who simply want to eat better and work less hard at it.

The senior author of this book, Dr. Sarah Morgan, shares with us important tips that show how in touch she is with individuals with arthritis. She is a physician who is a specialist in nutrition. She is a researcher who is a specialist in the role of nutrition and arthritis. Dr. Morgan is also a Registered Dietitian who knows how to translate the latest scientific research into easily understood, down-to-earth information that is useful for all readers. Working with a team of specialists in nutrition and arthritis, Dr. Morgan has brought us much more than a recipe book for people with arthritis. THE ESSENTIAL ARTHRITIS COOKBOOK is an important resource for anyone who wants to feel well and who is interested in good health through nutrition.

Roland L. Weinsier, M.D., Dr.P.H.
Professor and Chairman
Department of Nutrition Sciences
University of Alabama at Birmingham

From The Authors

As a physician trained in internal medicine and nutrition who sees patients with arthritis and does research in nutrition and arthritis, I have become impressed that nutrition does play a role in arthritis therapy. Maintenance of a healthy body weight as well as the nutrient content of foods consumed plays a role in the course of arthritis and other chronic diseases. We know that certain nutrients do have the capability to alter inflammation, and research in this area provides information for future treatments. I am often asked the questions like "What foods should I avoid or eat to make my arthritis better?" or "How do you expect me to cook and eat when my arthritis is bad?" These questions were the impetus for writing this book.

This source book, written by faculty members of the Department of Nutrition Sciences, the Multipurpose Arthritis and Musculoskeletal Disease Center and the Department of Occupational Therapy at the University of Alabama at Birmingham, has been written to provide basic nutrition information, information on kitchen planning and adaptive techniques, and recipes for people with arthritis and motion impairment. THE ESSENTIAL ARTHRITIS COOKBOOK takes your special needs into account — the recipes are easy to prepare; there are few ingredients; and there is minimal clean-up. Adaptive equipment, kitchen lay-out, time-saving and special meal preparation methods are suggested.

We hope that you will find this book educational and that it will provide you with new ideas to make your life easier. With a little knowledge, you can take control and cooking can be fun again.

Sarah L. Morgan, M.D., R.D., F.A.C.P.
Associate Professor of Medicine
Department of Nutrition Sciences
University of Alabama at Birmingham

Cooking used to be fun. It wasn't unusual for me to spend the morning in my kitchen, baking for friends, family, and myself. It was soothing to knead bread, knowing my time could be measured by the number of loaves I produced.

Then I was diagnosed with rheumatoid arthritis and just living each day became a challenge. Chronic pain and fatigue became my constant companions. Everyday activities became difficult to perform as the arthritis progressed and left me with more joint damage. Providing meals for myself and my family, however, continued to be important. I found myself surrendering to fast foods, convenience foods, and pizza delivery. I knew the importance of good nutrition, and I felt guilty that I could not provide my family with a healthy "home cooked" meal. In fact, I felt guilty about everything: that I had arthritis, that I couldn't do many activities and especially because my family could no longer depend on me for something as basic as food.

I felt out of control. Arthritis can be unpredictable, not only from day to day, but often from one hour to the next. I wanted more control in my life. I began to accept that I had a disease with no known cure and that there were some things that I would never be able to do again. But I am a strong believer in education and people. Working in the field of health education, I knew that I could not be the only person with arthritis who was having difficulty cooking. I also knew that if I had some nutrition knowledge and information about how to adapt cooking techniques for my unique needs that I would be able to regain some control.

I'm thrilled that this book gives me that control! THE ESSENTIAL ARTHRITIS COOKBOOK dispels many misconceptions surrounding arthritis and nutrition while providing so much practical information to help people with arthritis, like myself, minimize chronic pain and fatigue while working in the kitchen.

Janet Austin, M.Ed., Ph.D.
Director, Arthritis Information Service
University of Alabama at Birmingham

Introduction

Definition of Arthritis

The word arthritis means inflammation (redness, heat, swelling, tenderness) of the joints and is a general term used to describe over 100 diseases. Approximately 40 million Americans of all ages have arthritis, with the more serious forms commonly occuring between the ages of 20 and 50. This means that one in seven people and approximately one in three families are affected by arthritis. Women are affected twice as often as men. For the most part, arthritis lasts a lifetime. Some types of arthritis affect body parts outside the joints (for example skin rashes). In economic terms, arthritis is one of the nation's most disabling diseases and a leading cause of job absenteeism and disability payments.

The warning signs of arthritis are any of the following symptoms which persist for more than two weeks:

❑ Swelling in one or more joints

❑ Persistent early morning stiffness

❑ Recurring pain or tenderness in any joint

❑ Inability to move a joint normally

❑ Obvious redness and warmth in a joint

❑ Unexplained weight loss, fever, or decreased muscle strength combined with joint pain

The four most common types of arthritis are:

Osteoarthritis — "wear and tear arthritis"

Rheumatoid arthritis — an autoimmune arthritis (where the body attacks its own normal joint tissues)

Ankylosing spondylitis — spinal arthritis

Gout — a deposit of uric acid crystals in the joints

Only a physician can diagnose your specific type of arthritis. Other common types of arthritis-related disorders and syndromes include infectious arthritis, scleroderma, lupus, bursitis, tendonitis, fibromyalgia, and psoriatic arthritis.

Treatments for Arthritis

There are many treatments for arthritis which include rest, splinting of joints, exercise, occupational and physical therapy, a variety of medications and sometimes surgery. The medications most often used are nonsteroidal anti-inflammatory drugs including aspirin (NSAIDs), corticosteroids, gold, penicillamine, plaquenil, sulfasalazine, and other medications such as methotrexate, cytoxan, and immuran. A physician is the best person to diagnose and coordinate treatments of your arthritis. Nutrition is also an important treatment of arthritis. We have all heard the saying, "You are what you eat." Since foods are the building blocks of the body, it is not surprising that many diseases are caused or affected by what we eat. For example, eating too much fat is associated with obesity and aching joints. High blood pressure may be worsened in some people by consuming too much salt. General nutritional principles will be discussed in *Chapter 2* of this book.

Other Diseases that Cause Musculoskeletal Pain

Many other diseases cause musculoskeletal pain and fatigue but do not involve the joints. Fibromyalgia (fibrositis) and osteoporosis are other diseases which fit into this category.

Osteoporosis

Osteoporosis is a bone disease where there is an imbalance between bone formation and bone resorption, causing a reduction in bone mass. The ultimate and undesirable consequence of osteoporosis is bone fracture, often of the spine and hip. It is estimated that 26 million Americans are affected by osteoporosis; of these 20 million are women. The cost to our health care system is approximately $10 billion annually. Osteoporosis is diagnosed by dual-energy x-ray absorptiometry (DEXA). Osteoporosis must always be distinguished from other diseases causing low bone mass such as hyperthyroidism, Cushings syndrome, rheumatoid arthritis, and some cancers.

Risk Factors for Osteoporosis

Low peak bone mass: Peak bone mass is reached at approximately age 30. The higher the peak bone mass, the more bone may be lost before osteoporotic fractures occur.

Age and sex: Females are more at risk than males, particularly after menopause, when osteoporosis risk increases.

Heredity: Being Caucasian or Asiatic, of small stature, tall, lean, having long-term lactose intolerance, or a family history of osteoporosis puts an individual at higher risk for osteoporosis.

Nutrition: Chronic low calcium and vitamin D intakes can contribute to osteoporosis. Excessive intakes of sodium and protein can increase calcium losses in the urine making calcium from foods unavailable for the body to use.

Lifestyle habits: Cigarette smoking and heavy caffeine and alcohol intake are risk factors for osteoporosis. Excessive exercise in young women can predispose them to osteoporosis if it causes the cessation of menstrual periods. Regular weight-bearing exercise is helpful in preventing osteoporosis.

Medical factors: Many diseases such as rheumatoid arthritis and malabsorption can predispose an individual to low bone mass. Medications such as steroids (such as prednisone), excessive doses of thyroid hormone supplements and anticonvulsants often result in weaker bones when used for extended periods of time.

Fibromyalgia

Fibromyalgia or fibrositis is a syndrome where there is pain in the muscles and the fibrous connective tissues. Tender areas called trigger points are generally found on both sides of the body. The joints are not affected in fibromyalgia. Other symptoms that may occur in fibromyalgia include extreme fatigue, low exercise tolerance, altered sleep patterns, headaches (both migraines and tension headaches), and altered mood (anxiety and depression). The exact cause is unknown, and no one laboratory test can diagnose fibromyalgia. A careful medical history and physical examination should be done to rule out other causes of musculoskeletal pain.

The following chapters discuss how nutrition affects arthritis and other musculoskeletal diseases and translates the information into guidelines and recipes for good health.

Note: For more information on osteoporosis and fibromyalgia see *Chapter 1* and the *Recommended Reading List* at the end of that chapter.

Chapter 1:
Nutrition
and Arthritis

Contents

Chapter 1
NUTRITION AND ARTHRITIS

How Arthritis Can Affect Nutritional Status

Arthritis can affect the nutritional status of individuals in many ways. Morning stiffness may decrease appetite in the morning. Joint problems can interfere in the ability to shop, prepare, and eat foods. Arthritis in the jaws can affect chewing ability, and many of the drugs used to treat arthritis may cause nausea or diarrhea and have effects on nutrient absorption, metabolism, and bowel movements. All of these factors may place individuals with arthritis at a possible risk for nutrient deficiencies. It should also be realized that individuals with arthritis may be at risk for vitamin and mineral toxicity because of taking large amounts of vitamin and mineral preparations used as treatments or "curative" therapies.

Diet Treatment for Arthritis

What type of diet is best for the treatment of arthritis? First of all, **there is no specific "arthritis diet"** since there are so many specific types of arthritis. A well-balanced diet, as will be described in *Chapter 2*, is one that contains a variety of foods and is the best diet for good health for everyone. Therefore, fad diets which omit several foods or stress the benefits of a single food should be carefully evaluated. A diet containing plenty of fruits and vegetables, whole grain breads and cereals, and protein products (low-fat dairy foods, dried beans and peas, and lean meats) should be selected. Sweets (candies, cookies, pies, and cakes), fats and oils, snack foods (nuts and potato chips) and alcohol add extra calories and should be eaten in moderation.

Diet Therapy of Gout

Gouty arthritis is an example of a type of arthritis in which uric acid crystals are deposited within the joints and cause inflammation. While there are many drugs such as allopurinol and probenecid which are used in therapy for gout, dietary recommendations are important in preventing flare-ups.

Guidelines for gout therapy are outlined below:

* Healthy body weight should be maintained (see *Chapter 2 — Maintain a Healthy Weight*).

* If weight loss is necessary, gradual weight loss (1-2 pounds a week) is advisable. Fasting is detrimental because it increases blood uric acid levels.

* Because hypertriglyceridemia (elevated fats in the blood) often occur in people with gout, a diet low in fat, saturated fat, and cholesterol should be consumed (see *Chapter 2 — Choose A Diet Low in Total Fat, Saturated Fat, and Cholesterol*). In addition, people on high fat diets have decreased excretion of uric acid through the kidneys, causing higher blood levels of uric acid.

* Alcohol increases blood uric acid levels, therefore alcohol, especially beer, should be consumed in moderation or not at all.

* Liberal amounts of fluid (2-3 quarts a day) should be consumed to help with uric acid excretion and to prevent uric acid kidney stones.

* Because protein foods contain purines, from which uric acid is produced, protein intake should be limited to 4-6 ounces of meat, fish, or poultry a day (about the size of 2 decks of cards), to prevent excessive uric acid production (see *Chapter 2*).

Dietary purines are the precursors of uric acid in the body. The guidelines listed above are the best nutritional advice for patients with gouty arthritis. Foods that are high or low in purines are listed on the next page.

Table 1:	
Foods Low in Purines	**Foods High in Purines**
Fruits	Sweetbreads
Fruit juices	(thymus glands from selected animals)
Vegetables (except	Anchovies
dried beans and peas, lentils,	Herring
asparagus, cauliflower, spinach,	Mackerel
peas, and mushrooms)	Scallops
Milk	Sardines
Cheese	Liver
Eggs	Kidney
Breads, cereals and pasta	Red meat and meat extracts
(except whole grain bread products and oatmeal)	Wild game
Coffee	Chicken, turkey and goose
Tea	Dried beans and peas
Carbonated beverages	Lentils
Gelatin	Asparagus, cauliflower, spinach
Nuts	Mushrooms

Obesity and Osteoarthritis

The prevention and treatment of obesity is important for osteoarthritis. Several studies have supported an association between obesity and "wear and tear" arthritis on weight-bearing joints, particularly the knees. However, the relationship is complicated because osteoarthritis also occurs in nonweight-bearing joints in people who are overweight. Osteoarthritis has many causes, but the association between fat tissue and arthritis in some weight-bearing joints is strong. Therefore, weight reduction and the maintenance of a healthy body weight are important considerations. Maintaining a healthy body weight is also important for the prevention of other conditions such as heart disease and will be discussed in *Chapter 2*.

Fad Diets and Arthritis

Patients with arthritis often turn to a variety of unproven remedies and fad diets. Unproven remedies may be spotted by using the checklist provided by the Arthritis Foundation which is shown on this and the next page. Many fad diets are promoted as remedies but are unproven. These diets often emphasize eating specific foods or eliminating specific foods or groups of foods. Diets may promote certain foods such as apple cider and honey, brewer's yeast, wheat germ, pokeweed berries, garlic, cod liver oil, alfalfa, and blackstrap molasses. If the checklist for unproven remedies is used for the previous suggested therapies, you can see that they are **not** valuable therapies for arthritis therapy. An emphasis on a specific food can cause a diet to be unbalanced, with the possibility of vitamin and mineral deficiencies.

A variety of diet plans have been suggested including the elimination of acidic fruits and vegetables and low protein diets. The Dong Diet, which is free of additives, preservatives, fruit, red meat, herbs and dairy products was studied by Dr. Richard Panush in a placebo-controlled, double-blind trial.[1] He was not able to demonstrate any clinical benefits from the diet in a large group of patients. In summary, many diets that are publicized for arthritis therapy are not supported by science and may cause malnutrition. A registered/licensed dietitian or your physician is the best source for information regarding the safety of such diets.

Checklist For Spotting an Unproven Remedy

IS IT LIKELY TO WORK FOR ME?
Suspect an unproven remedy if it:

❑ Claims to work for all types of arthritis as well as other health problems

❑ Uses only case histories or testimonials as proof

❑ Cites only one study as proof

❑ Cites a study without a control group

HOW SAFE IS IT?
Suspect an unproven remedy if it:

❑ Comes without any directions for proper use

❑ Does not list contents

❑ Has no information or warning about side effects

❑ Is described as harmless or natural

HOW IS IT PROMOTED?
Suspect an unproven remedy if it:

❑ Claims it's based on a secret formula

❑ Claims it cures arthritis

❑ Is available only from one source

❑ Is promoted only in the media, books, or by mail order

Excerpted with permission from Unproven Remedies, copyright 1987 by the Arthritis Foundation. For further information or for a complete copy of this booklet, write the Arthritis Foundation, PO Box 19000, Atlanta GA 30326, or contact your local chapter.

The Use of Single Nutrients in the Treatment of Arthritis

Deficiencies of a variety of vitamins and minerals have been documented in individual patients with certain types of arthritis. Some of the nutrients which have attracted interest include zinc, selenium, and vitamin C. However, there are no vitamin or mineral deficiencies which are characteristic of a person with a certain type of arthritis. Therefore, attempts to treat a type of arthritis with massive doses of a single vitamin or mineral have not been proven to be useful. Many nutritional supplements which are sold as essential nutrients such as bioflavenoids, in reality are not essential for humans. Vitamin supplementation, especially doses which are 5 to 10 times above the daily value for a nutrient (see *Appendix B* for a discussion of daily values) should be monitored by a physician. Toxicity syndromes for both fat and water soluble vitamins exist. Therefore, taking vitamin and mineral supplements is not always without risk. The decision to use a vitamin or mineral supplement as an arthritis treatment should be made after consulting with the physician caring for your arthritis. If general vitamin/mineral supplementation is desired, a vitamin which provides 100% of the Daily Values for vitamins and minerals is a reasonable choice, and one vitamin capsule a day should be taken (for example Centrum®, Unicaps®, One-A-Day®).

Diet and Immune Function

The immune system of the body is composed of both cells and substances in the blood and is the natural defense against infections and cancer. The immune system is activated in some forms of arthritis to produce inflammation in the joints. Dietary components and the immune system are linked. Nutrients can affect the immune response and there is concern that food substances can produce immune-regulated reactions that may be a cause of some forms of arthritis, like rheumatoid arthritis.

Food Allergies and Arthritis

Food allergy is a term which describes a reaction to foods in which the immune system is involved. There is a theory that substances in foods that are absorbed through the intestine may be involved in starting the inflammatory response. True food allergies may cause an allergic reaction called anaphylaxis and have skin, lung, or bowel-related symptoms. Double-blind food challenge tests can be used to document true food allergies. These tests evaluate the response to foods when neither the researcher nor the study participant knows what the participant is receiving (i.e. food or nonfood). Corn, wheat, pork, oranges, milk, oats, rye, eggs, and beef have been suggested to be the foods most likely related to allergic arthritis. However, it is estimated that **less than 5% of immune-related arthritis is related to food allergies**. If a specific food causes your arthritis to worsen, then it is probably safe to omit that one food from your diet. Groups of foods (i.e. all fruits, all vegetables) should **not** be omitted from the diet because this could lead to an unbalanced diet and malnutrition. The advice of your physician and registered/licensed dietitian can be helpful in making dietary changes.

Fish Oils and Arthritis:
Possible Benefits and Dangers

Nutrients have been identified which decrease inflammation and therefore lessen joint symptoms. Prostaglandins are produced from fatty acids in cell membranes which can alter inflammation in the body. The type of prostaglandins synthesized can be influenced by the kind of dietary fat consumed. Omega-3 fatty acids are a special type of fatty acid found in cold water fish. A study done by Dr. Joel Kremer evaluated patients with rheumatoid arthritis given fish oil tablets (omega-3 fatty acids) for up to 24 weeks. The patients on fish oil had fewer tender and swollen joints and less morning stiffness than patients treated with olive oil capsules. Dr. Kremer was able to document that substances with less inflammatory activity were produced in the fish oil-treated subjects, thereby contributing to less joint inflammation.[2] Numerous other studies have confirmed these findings.

However, the optimal dose in treating rheumatoid arthritis and the long term effects of omega-3 fatty acid supplementation are not known. Additionally, the cost of omega-3 fatty acid capsules can be quite expensive. **There are also potential side effects from fish oil consumption.** If large amounts of omega-3 fatty acids are consumed as cod liver oil, there is a risk of vitamin A and vitamin D toxicity. Large amounts of fish oil can also add calories to the diet with the risk of weight gain. Omega-3 fatty acids also impair the ability of blood clotting cells known as platelets to work. Preliminary studies in rats fed omega-3 fatty acids show changes in joint cartilage cells consistent with early osteoarthrosis, but that effect has not been found or studied in humans. The decision to take omega-3 fatty acids should be done with the guidance of a physician. A reasonable recommendation is to consume fish two to three times a week rather than relying upon supplements. Individuals who should not take fish oil supplements include children, adolescents, pregnant women, individuals with bleeding disorders, and individuals on blood thinners (such as Coumadin® and Warfarin). In addition, patients with serious medical disorders, on multiple medications, should always discuss taking fish oil capsules with their physician before beginning such therapy. All seafood contains omega-3 fatty acids, however, cold water fish and fish with a higher fat content are the best sources of omega-3 fatty acids.

Table 2: Fish High in Omega -3 Fatty Acids
 (more than 1 gram per 3 1/2 ounces raw)

Salmon	Sardines
Herring	Rainbow trout
Bluefish	Lake trout
Tuna	Lake whitefish
Mackerel	Anchovy
Spiny dogfish	Sablefish

from SEAFOOD AND HEALTH by Joyce Nettleton. Osprey Books, 1987. See also Recommended Reading List.

Fasting and Vegetarian Diets in the Treatment of Rheumatoid Arthritis

It has been a part of nutritional folklore that fasting is a useful therapy for the treatment of rheumatoid arthritis. Several studies have recently evaluated the effects of fasting followed by a vegetarian diet on arthritis. Vegetarian diets can be classified as vegan (no animal products), lactovegetarian (includes dairy products), ovovegetarian (includes egg products) and pescovegetarian (includes fish). There can also be various combinations of the above vegetarian diets.

Dr. Lars Skoldstam in Sweden studied patients with rheumatoid arthritis who fasted for 7 to 10 days and then were randomized to receive either a regular diet or a vegan (no animal products) or a lactovegetarian diet (milk products allowed).[3] The investigator noted improvements in stiffness and pain after 7 to 10 days of fasting. The vegetarian diet had no objective effects on disease activity in either of the studies.[4]

A study in *The Lancet* in 1991 compared 27 patients who stayed for 4 weeks at a health farm and underwent a 7 to 10 day fast followed by a vegetarian diet for 1 year with 26 patients staying at a convalescent home for 4 weeks followed by a normal diet. The patients on the vegetarian diet lost more weight than the control group and had significant improvements in the pain/tenderness and swelling of their joints after 1 year compared to the control group. However, this study was criticized because it was felt that the subjects were not randomly selected and that a high percentage of the study subjects had food allergies which complicated the interpretation of the study.[5]

It does seem clear that fasting has a beneficial effect on rheumatoid arthritis. However, as a treatment it is not a practical one since long-term fasting can lead to dehydration, nutrient deficiencies, and ultimately death. The effects of a vegetarian diet on rheumatoid arthritis activity are controversial. The reported response of study patients reported in *The Lancet* may have been due to a placebo response, suppression of immune-related reactions, or changes in the permeability of the gastrointestinal tract. The hypothesis about the gastrointestinal tract is an interesting one. It has been suggested that many of the drugs used to treat arthritis may cause the intestine to be "leaky" and allow foods and bacteria to pass through, which may contribute to an increased immune response and inflammation.

Therefore, the use of a vegetarian diet needs to be further studied before it can be established as an accepted treatment for rheumatoid arthritis. However, vegetarian diets can have a number of benefits since they are generally high in fiber, low in fat, saturated fat, and cholesterol and can be conducive to weight loss when compared to the average American diet. If a vegetarian diet pattern is selected, it is important to eat a wide variety of foods, since it is still necessary to meet the daily requirements for vitamins, minerals, fluid, and protein. A registered/licensed dietitian can help you evaluate the adequacy of a vegetarian meal pattern.

Nutritional Therapies for Osteoporosis and Fibromyalgia

Osteoporosis

Adequate calcium and vitamin D intake is important in prevention and treatment of osteoporosis. The following amounts of calcium are recommended by the National Institutes of Health Consensus Panel[6]:

Table 3: Calcium Recommendations

Children, ages 1-5	800 mg/day
Children, ages 6-10	800-1200 mg/day
Adolescents, ages 11-24	1200-1500 mg/day
Women, ages 25-50	1000 mg/day
Women, pregnant and nursing	1200-1500mg/day

Postmenopausal Women over 50 not on estrogen	1500 mg/day
Postmenopausal Women over 50 on estrogen	1000 mg/day
Women over 65	1500mg/day
Men, ages 25-65	1000 mg/day
Men over 65	1500 mg/day

Following the Food Guide Pyramid guidelines (see **Chapter 2**) can assure that reasonable amounts of sodium and protein are consumed so as not to interfere with calcium absorption.

Vitamin D is formed in the skin from exposure to sunlight and found in fortified milk products. The Recommended Daily Value for vitamin D is 400 International Units a day. Vitamin D is important in helping the body absorb calcium, and a variety of vitamin D products can be used to treat osteoporosis.

Other important therapies for prevention and treatment of osteoporosis include avoiding tobacco, excessive alcohol and caffeine intake, and moderate weight-bearing exercise. Hormone replacement, calcitonin and biophosphonate therapies can also be useful in the treatment of osteoporosis.

Fibromyalgia

Following the Food Guide Pyramid guidelines (see **Chapter 2**) is the best dietary approach for the treatment of fibromyalgia. Attaining or maintaining a reasonable body weight may also be useful in patients with fibromyalgia. Narcotic pain relievers and steroid drugs (such as prednisone) should be avoided. Medications that aid sleep and relax muscles may be useful, and exercise, both gentle aerobics and aquatic, is often recommended.

Arthritis Medications and Diet

Many arthritis medications affect vitamin and mineral levels in the body by affecting absorption, changing metabolism or increasing losses of the nutrient from the body. The table on the following page lists some of the drugs used for the treatment of arthritis, their pronunciations, brand names, and their uses.

Table 4: Arthritis Medications

Name	Pronunciation	Brand Name	Common Use
Nonsteroidal Anti-inflammatory Drugs	non-stare-OID-al		Anti-inflammatory
Aspirin	AS-pi-rin	Bayer, Anacin	Anti-inflammatory
Ibuprofen	ie-byu-PROE-fin	Advil, Medipren, Motrin, Nuprin, Rufen, Arthritis Foundation	Anti-inflammatory
Naproxen	na-PROCKS-in	Anaprox, Naprosyn, Aleve	Anti-inflammatory
Indomethacin	in-doe-METH-a-sin	Indocin	Anti-inflammatory
Sulindac	sue-LIN-dak	Clinoril	Anti-inflammatory
Tolmetin	TOEL-me-tin	Tolectin	Anti-inflammatory
Piroxicam	peer-OCKS-i-kam	Feldene	Anti-inflammatory
Nabumetone	na-BYU-me-tone	Relafen	Anti-inflammatory
Etodolac	e-toe-DOE-lak	Lodine	Anti-inflammatory
Meclofenamate	mek-loe-FEN-a-mate	Meclomen	Anti-inflammatory
Diflunisal	die-FLUE-ni-sal	Dolobid	Anti-inflammatory
Ketorolac	ket-oe-ROEL-ak	Toradol	Anti-inflammatory
Prednisone	PRED-ni-sone	Deltasone	Anti-inflammatory

Table 4: Arthritis Medications continued

Name	Pronunciation	Brand Name	Common Use
Acetominophen	a-seat-a-MIN-a fen	Tylenol	Pain reliever
Penicillamine	pen-i-SIL-a-meen	Cuprimine, Depen Titratable Tablets	Rheumatoid arthritis medication
Hydroxy-chloroquine	hi-drock-see-KLOR-o-kwin	Plaquenil	Rheumatoid arthritis medication
Gold salts	gold salts		Rheumatoid arthritis medication
Methotrexate	meth-o-TRECK-sate	Rheumatrex, Mexate	Rheumatoid arthritis medication
Sulfasalazine	sul-fah-SAL-ah-zeen	Azulfidine	Rheumatoid arthritis medication
Allopurinol	al-o-PURE-in-ahl	Zyloprim	Antigout
Probenecid	proe-BEN-i-sid	Benemid	Antigout
Colchicine	KOL-chi-sin	Colbenemide	Antigout

Arthritis Medication and Nutrition

Definitive studies have generally not been done to determine how much more of these specific nutrients are necessary while taking a specific drug for arthritis. The best advice is to consume at least the Recommend Daily Value for these nutrients. The table on the next page lists the Recommended Daily Value for nutrients discussed in this section. Your physician is the best guide whether additional supplements are necessary. *Appendix B* discusses using food labels to help you consume 100% of the Recommended Daily Values for nutrients daily.

Table 5: Recommended Daily Values

Nutrient	100% of the Reference Daily Intake
Vitamin B_6	2.0 milligrams
Vitamin B_{12}	6 micrograms
Vitamin C	60 milligrams
Vitamin D	400 International Units
Vitamin K	RDI not established
Folic Acid	0.4 milligrams
Calcium	1000 milligrams
Copper	2 milligrams
Iron	18 milligrams
Magnesium	400 milligrams
Phosphorus	1000 milligrams
Potassium	4000 milligrams
Sodium	2400 milligrams
Zinc	15 milligrams

Aspirin and nonsteroidal anti-inflammatory drugs, commonly used for all types of arthritis, can cause stomach or intestinal bleeding which can increase iron and folic acid needs. Eating foods high in iron and folic acid can help meet increased needs.

Table 6:

Good Sources of Iron	Good Sources of Folic Acid
Liver	Grapefruit and orange juice
Lean red meat and poultry	Green leafy vegetables
Dried fruits	Asparagus
Dried beans, lentils	Broccoli
Clams, oysters, sardines	Fortified cereals
Tofu	Dried beans and peas
Enriched breads and cereals	Liver and other organ meats
Green leafy vegetables	Cantaloupe

Aspirin may also increase vitamin C losses from the body. Good sources of vitamin C are listed in the table on the next page.

Table 7: Good Sources of Vitamin C

Green peppers	Broccoli	Cabbage	Brussels sprouts
Grapefruit	Potatoes	Tomatoes	Strawberries
Oranges	Papayas	Cantaloupe	Lemons
Honeydew melon	Limes	Tangerines	Asparagus
Cauliflower	Mangos	Kiwi fruit	Sweet potatoes
Fortified juices	Green leafy vegetables		

Colchicine is a drug used in the treatment of gout. If taken in high doses, it can cause damage to the lining of the intestine and cause poor absorption of fat, sodium, potassium, calcium, phosphorus, magnesium, vitamin B_{12}, vitamin D, and vitamin K. Generally, since colchicine is only used in high doses for very short periods of time, this should not be a major problem. Your physician is aware of these interactions and will discontinue the drug before malabsorption occurs. These side effects are reversed 4-7 days after stopping the drug. The following tables list good sources of vitamin B_{12}, vitamin D, vitamin K, magnesium, potassium, and phosphorus. (See Table 14 for a list of good sources of calcium.)

Table 8: Good Sources of Vitamin B_{12}

All foods of **animal origin** contain vitamin B_{12}

Lean meats, fish, and poultry	Eggs (Limit to 3-4 yolks/week)
Low-fat milk and milk products	

Table 9:

Good Sources of Vitamin D	**Good Sources of Vitamin K**
Herring	Beef liver
Salmon	Cauliflower, broccoli, cabbage
Fortified milk	Brussel sprouts, asparagus
Liver	Spinach, lettuce
Shrimp	Kale/other green leafy vegetables
Egg yolks	Turnip greens
	Peaches
	Cheese

Table 10: Good Sources of Potassium

Lean meat, fish, and poultry	Asparagus
Nonfat yogurt	Green leafy vegetables
Watermelon	Baked potatoes
Oranges and orange juice	Dried beans and peas
Prunes, raisins and dates	Cauliflower
Cantaloupe	Tomatoes
Bananas	Broccoli
Dried apricots and peaches	Whole grains

Table 11:

Good Sources of Phosphorus	Good Sources of Magnesium
Lean meats, fish, and poultry	Whole grain breads and cereals
Low-fat milk	Dried beans and peas
Low-fat cheese	Broccoli
Peanuts	Spinach
Dried beans and peas	Oysters, scallops
Soft drinks	Nuts and seeds
	Low-fat milk
	Tofu

Methotrexate and sulfasalazine are used particularly for rheumatoid arthritis therapy and act against folic acid, a B-vitamin. Your physician may decide to give you folic acid supplements if you are taking these medications. There is evidence that eating at least 100% of the Daily Recommended Value of folic acid, while taking low-dose methotrexate for rheumatoid arthritis, can help to lower the toxicity of methotrexate. Recent experiments have demonstrated that 5, 7, or 27.5 mg of supplemental folic acid weekly lowered methotrexate toxicity without affecting drug activity.[7] Foods which are good sources of folic acid have been previously listed.

D-penicillamine binds to various minerals such as copper, zinc, iron and vitamin B6 (pyridoxine), which can reduce the absorption of these minerals. Foods high in zinc, copper, and vitamin B6 are listed on the next page.

Table 12:

Good Sources of Zinc	Good Sources of Copper
Oysters	Lobster
Lean meats	Oysters
Eggs	Barley
Green peas	Prunes
Barley	Dried beans and peas
Whole wheat bread	Nuts
Liver	Beef and calf liver

Table 13: Good Sources of B$_6$ (Pyridoxine)

Salmon	Lean poultry
Lean beef	Tuna, packed in water
Potatoes	Bananas
Brewer's Yeast	
Liver	

Corticosteroids, such as prednisone, are widely used to treat a variety of arthritis-related conditions. Corticosteroids can cause salt and water retention which can cause edema (fluid retention). Corticosteroids also lower calcium absorption, and alter vitamin D metabolism. Following a low sodium (salt) diet, while obtaining adequate vitamin D, calcium, and phosphorus is helpful. It is important to note that many low sodium and reduced-sodium products are now available at the supermarket (see more information on labeling in *Appendix B*). Most rheumatologists recommend that individuals on steroids consume at least 1000-1500 mg of calcium a day (see Consensus Panel recommendations for calcium intake, Table 3).

Table 14: Good Sources of Calcium

Low-fat milk	Low-fat cheese
Nonfat yogurt	Fat-free ice cream
Green leafy vegetables	Salmon canned with bones

Table 15: A Sodium-Restricted Diet

Item	Foods Low in Sodium	Foods to Limit
Beverages	Coffee, tea, unsoftened water	Buttermilk
Breads	Unsalted breads and crackers	Salted breads and crackers
Protein Foods	Noncured beef, pork, veal, lamb, chicken, and turkey	Ham, corned beef, hot dogs, luncheon meats, canned salmon and tuna, cheese
Soups	Low-sodium soups Low-sodium bouillon	Regular soups, bouillon, consommé
Vegetables	Fresh vegetables, low-sodium vegetable juices, low-sodium canned vegetables	Sauerkraut, regular canned vegetables, or vegetable juices
Fruits	All fruits	None
Fats	Low-sodium peanut butter, gravy made without added salt or bouillon, unsalted nuts	Peanut butter gravies, bacon, salted nuts
Miscellaneous	Pepper, salt-free seasoning mixtures such as lemon pepper, Mrs. Dash® , low-sodium soy sauce and Worcestershire sauce, unsalted popcorn, pretzels, and snacks	Salt, seasoned salts, monosodium glutamate (MSG), Kitchen Bouquet®,Worcestershire sauce, steak sauces, teriyaki sauce, soy sauce, catsup, mustard, pickles, olives, salted snack foods

Many drugs taken to reduce nausea caused by arthritis medications can also alter nutrient balance. The regular use of aluminum- and magnesium-containing antacids can lower phosphorus absorption. Good sources of phosphorus are listed in the discussion regarding colchicine.

SUMMARY

In summary, there is no special "arthritis diet" or special diet for musculoskeletal diseases. Consuming foods using the Food Guide Pyramid (see *Chapter 2*) is the best recommendation. Research shows that certain nutrients do affect inflammation and immune status. At the present time, obtaining those nutrients from a wide variety of foods is the best strategy.

Toll Free Numbers to Call About Nutrition and Arthritis/Musculoskeletal Diseases

* American Lupus Society, 1-800-331-1802.
* Ankylosing Spondylitis Association, 1-800-777-8189.
* Arthritis Foundation Information Line, 1-800-283-7800.
* Lupus Foundation of America, 1-800-558-0121.
* The Arthritis Information Service, The University of Alabama at Birmingham, 1-800-345-6780.
* The Calcium Information Center, a service of Oregon Health Sciences University and Cornell Medical Center, 1-800-321-2681.
* The National Center for Nutrition and Dietetics, the America Dietetic Association, Chicago, Illinois, 1-800-366-1655.
* The Nutrition Information Service, The University of Alabama at Birmingham, 1-800-231-3438.
* United Scleroderma Foundation, 1-800-722-HOPE.

Works Cited

[1]Panush, Richard, et al. "Dietary Therapy for Rheumatoid Arthritis." ARTHRITIS AND RHEUMATISM 26/4 (April 1983): 462-471.

[2]Kremer, Joel, et al. "Dietary fish oil and olive oil supplementation in patients with rheumatoid arthritis. Clinical and immunological effects." ARTHRITIS AND RHEUMATISM 33/6 (June 1990): 810-820.

[3]Skoldstam, Lars, et al. "Effect of Fasting and Lactovegetarian Diet on Rheumatoid Arthritis." SCANDINAVIAN JOURNAL OF RHEUMATOLOGY 8/4 (1979): 249-255.

[4]Skoldstam, Lars, et al. "Fasting and Vegan Diet in Rheumatoid Arthritis." SCANDINAVIAN JOURNAL OF RHEUMATOLOGY 15/2 (1986): 219-221.

[5]Kjeldsen-Krogh, J, et al. "Controlled Trial and Fasting and One-Year Vegetarian Diet in Rheumatoid Arthritis." LANCET 338/8772 (12 October 1991): 899-902.

[6]NIH Consensus Development Panel on Optimal Calcium Intake. JOURNAL AMERICAN MEDICAL ASSOCIATION. 272(1994):1942-1948.

[7]Morgan, Sarah, et al. "Supplementation with Folic Acid During Methotrexate Therapy for Rheumatoid Arthritis. A Double-Blind Controlled Trial." ANNALS OF INTERNAL MEDICINE 121 (1994): 833-841.

For Further Reading

Dietary Intakes of Patients with Arthritis and the Effect of Diet on Arthritis

ARTHRITIS AND RHEUMATISM. "Food-induced (allergic) arthritis. Inflammatory arthritis exacerbated by milk," by R. Panush, et al. 1986. 29(2):220-226.

ARTHRITIS CARE AND RESEARCH. "Dietary intake and circulating vitamin levels of rheumatoid arthritis patients treated with methotrexate," by S. Morgan, et al. 1993. 6(1):4-10.

ARTHRITIS CARE AND RESEARCH. "Dietary and allergic associations with rheumatoid arthritis. Self-Report of 704 patients," by S.B. Tanner, et al. 1990.

BRITISH JOURNAL OF RHEUMATOLOGY. "Is diet important in rheumatoid arthritis?" by H. M. Buchanan, et, al. 1991. 30(2):125-34.

CLINICAL RHEUMATOLOGY. "Malnutrition in rheumatoid adults," by R. Collins, et al. 1987. 6(3):391-398.

JOURNAL OF THE AMERICAN DIETETIC ASSOCIATION. "Nutritional considerations in rheumatoid arthritis," by R. Tougher-Decker. 1988.88(3): 327-331.

JOURNAL OF THE AMERICAN DIETETIC ASSOCIATION. "Assessment of the diet
of patients with rheumatoid arthritis and osteoarthritis," by B. Kowsari. 1983.
82(6):657-659.
NUTRITION AND RHEUMATIC DISEASES. Dietary therapy for arthritis," by L.G.
Darlington. 1991. 17(2):273-284

Diet and Nutrient Interactions

ARTHRITIS AND RHEUMATISM. "Folate status of rheumatoid arthritis patients
receiving long-term, low-dose methotrexate therapy," by S. Morgan, et al.
1987. 30:1348-1356.
ARTHRITIS AND RHEUMATISM. "The effect of folic acid supplementation on the
toxicity of low-dose methotrexate in patients with rheumatoid arthritis," by
S. Morgan, et al. 1990. 33(1):9-18.
BIOCHEMICAL JOURNAL. "Inhibition of folate-dependent enzymes by nonsteroidal
anti-inflammatory drugs," by J. E. Baggott. 1992. 282(pt 1):197-202.

Fad Diets

ARTHRITIS UNPROVEN REMEDIES. The Arthritis Foundation. 1987.
ARTHRITIS AND RHEUMATISM. "The Unproven Remedies Committee," by M.
Lockshin. 1981. 24(9):1188-1190.

Fasting and Vegetarian Diets and Arthritis

CLINICAL RHEUMATOLOGY. "The influence of fasting and vegetarian diet on
parameters of nutritional status in patients with rheumatoid arthritis," by M. A.
Haugen, et al. 1993. 12(1):62-69.

Fibromyalgia

PRIMER ON RHEUMATIC DISEASES, by R. Schumacher, et al. Arthritis
Foundation, 1988.

Fish Oil and Arthritis

ANNALS OF INTERNAL MEDICINE. "Fish-oil fatty acid supplementation in active
rheumatoid arthritis," by J.M. Kremer, et al. 1987. 106:497-503.
ARTHRITIS AND RHEUMATISM. "Metabolic and ultrastructural changes in articular
cartilage of rats fed dietary supplements of omega-3 fatty acids," by L. Lippiello,
M. Fienhold, C. Grandjean. 1990. 33(7):1029-1036.
ARTHRITIS AND RHEUMATISM. "Dietary fish oil and olive oil supplementation in
patients with rheumatoid arthritis," by J. M. Kremer, et al. 1990. 33(6):810-820.
JOURNAL OF THE AMERICAN MEDICAL ASSOCIATION. "Clinical applications of
fish oils," by J. Z. Yetiv. 1988. 260(5):665-670.
SEAFOOD AND HEALTH by J. Nettleton. Osprey Books, 1987.

Food Allergies

ANNALS OF THE RHEUMATIC DISEASES. "Food intolerance in rheumatoid arthritis. I. A double-blind, controlled trial of the clinical effects of elimination of milk allergens and azo dyes," by M. van de Laar and J. van der Korst. 1992. 51(3):298-302.

ARTHRITIS AND RHEUMATISM. "Dietary Therapy for Rheumatoid Arthritis," by R. Panush, et al. 1983. 26(4):462-471.

ANNALS OF THE RHEUMATIC DISEASES. "Food intolerance in rheumatoid arthritis. II. Clinical and histological aspects," by M. van de Laar. 51(3):303-306.

Gout

MANUAL FOR NUTRITIONAL MANAGEMENT by Department of Food and Nutrition. University of Alabama-Birmingham, 1993.

RECENT ADVANCES IN THERAPEUTIC DIETS by Dietary Department. University of Iowa Hospitals and Clinics/Iowa State University Press, 1989.

LANCET. "Effect of weight-loss on plasma and urinary levels of uric acid," by A. Nicholls and J.T. Scott. 1972. 2(789):1123-1224.

Obesity and Osteoarthritis

ANNALS OF THE RHEUMATIC DISEASES. "New Haven survey of joint diseases. XVII. Relationship between some systemic characteristics and osteoporosis in a general population," by R.M. Acheson and A.B. Collart. October 1975. 34(5):379-387.

JOURNAL OF THE AMERICAN COLLEGE OF NUTRITION. "Rational Weight Loss Programs: A Clinician's Guide," by S. Morgan. June 1989. 8(3):186-194.

THE JOURNAL OF RHEUMATOLOGY. "Osteoporosis and obesity in the general population. A relationship calling for an explanation," by J. van Saase. 1988. 15(7):1152.

Osteoporosis

JOURNAL OF THE AMERICAN MEDICAL ASSOCIATION. "Optimal calcium intake," by National Consensus Conference. 1994. 15(7):1942-1947.

PRIMER ON METABOLIC BONE DISEASES AND DISORDERS OF MINERAL METABOLISM, 2nd edition, by M. J. Farvus. Raven Press, 1993.

Chapter 2:
Basic
Nutrition

Contents

Chapter 2
BASIC NUTRITION

Quality of Life

There is no magical "arthritis diet." However, consuming a healthy balanced diet is one of the most important things you can do to help your arthritis. Preventing disability and treating chronic diseases, including arthritis, depends on individual decisions — to consume less fat and sodium; to consume more fiber; to increase physical activity; to drink alcohol in moderation, if at all; to control weight and caloric intake; to control stress — in other words, to take control of our lives.

One measure of health that considers quality of life as well as length of life is the years of healthy life. Another indicator of quality of life is an individual's ability to perform activities required for daily living, such as cooking and eating. The challenge facing each of us is to maintain our health and prevent disease. Our individual decisions are affected by many things. Good nutrition habits are one of the choices we can make towards keeping or improving health.

The Dietary Guidelines for Americans

The Dietary Guidelines for Americans, which are listed in the following pages, can serve as a useful outline for choosing a healthy, balanced diet while decreasing the risk of developing chronic diseases such as cancer and heart disease. They are recommended for everyone age 2 and up and can even be modified to be used by persons on special diets prescribed by their physicians. The recipes in this cookbook were developed to help an individual easily prepare meals, while still meeting the goals set by the Dietary Guidelines for Americans. The Food Guide Pyramid is a visual representation of the Dietary Guidelines for Americans.

Food Guide Pyramid

A Guide to Daily Food Choices

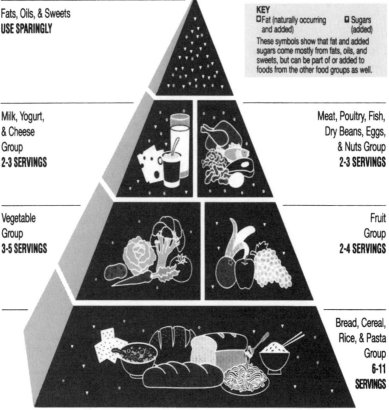

Fats, Oils, & Sweets
USE SPARINGLY

KEY
☐ Fat (naturally occurring   ▨ Sugars
and added)   (added)
These symbols show that fat and added
sugars come mostly from fats, oils, and
sweets, but can be part of or added to
foods from the other food groups as well.

Milk, Yogurt,
& Cheese
Group
2-3 SERVINGS

Meat, Poultry, Fish,
Dry Beans, Eggs,
& Nuts Group
2-3 SERVINGS

Vegetable
Group
3-5 SERVINGS

Fruit
Group
2-4 SERVINGS

Bread, Cereal,
Rice, & Pasta
Group
**6-11
SERVINGS**

SOURCE: U.S. Department of Agriculture/U.S. Department of Health and Human Services

Food Guide Pyramid. Source: USDA and USDHHS

Nutrition and Your Health:
Dietary Guidelines for Americans

* Eat a variety of foods.

* Maintain a healthy weight.

* Choose a diet low in fat, saturated fat, and cholesterol.

* Choose a diet with plenty of vegetables, fruits, and grain products.

* Use sugars only in moderation.

* Use salt and sodium only in moderation.

* If you drink alcoholic beverages, do so in moderation.

Source: USDA and USDHHS, 3rd Edition, 1990 (Home and Garden Bulletin No. 232).

Eat a Variety of Foods

The Dietary Guidelines stress the importance of eating a variety of low-fat foods, including fruits and vegetables and grain products. By selecting a wide variety of foods, it is possible to have an adequate intake of vitamins, minerals, fat, protein, and carbohydrate.

This means a number of different foods should be eaten in order to meet nutritional requirements for vitamins, minerals, carbohydrates, fats, and proteins. For the rest of this book, these will be referred to as *nutrients*. These nutrients should not be obtained solely from supplements or enriched foods. For example, calcium is more absorbable when obtained from dairy foods than from calcium supplements. Calcium is an important nutrient that has been shown to decrease risk for osteoporosis. Therefore, getting a balanced diet which includes dairy products is important. Any food can be part of a nutritious diet. It is the nutritional balance achieved over days and weeks of healthy eating that makes a difference.

How Do I Know If I Am Eating a Balanced Diet?

Another way to visualize good eating is by looking at the Food Guide Pyramid. Foods at the base of the pyramid should be eaten more frequently.

The recommended number of daily servings of different foods for adults is as follows (see the Food Guide Pyramid):

Breads, cereals, grains and pasta:	6-11 servings
Fruits:	2-4 servings
Vegetables:	3-5 servings
Meat, poultry, fish, and legumes:	2-3 servings
Dairy:	2-3 servings
Fats, oils and sweets	Use sparingly

Examples of one serving of a food are defined as follows:

Breads, Cereals, Grains, and Cereals:
1 slice of bread or 1/2 cup of rice or pasta, 1 ounce ready-to-eat cereal

Fruits:
1 medium piece of fruit or 3/4 cup fruit juice, 1/4 cup dried fruit

Vegetables:
1/2 cup cooked or chopped raw vegetables, 1 cup leafy raw vegetables

Meat:
2 1/2-3 ounces of meat, poultry, or fish is the amount equivalent to the size of one deck of playing cards. One egg counts as 1 ounce of meat.

Dairy:
1 cup of low-fat milk or low-fat yogurt, 1 1/2 ounces of low-fat cheese

Keeping a record of the foods you eat is a good way to check if you are eating a variety of foods and therefore a balanced diet. This is an example of the daily food intake of a person with an analysis of the variety of foods eaten.

Table 16: Sample Food Intake

Breakfast:
One poached egg
1 square CINNAMON COFFEE CAKE (page 205)
Grapefruit half
1 cup of skim milk

Lunch:
Cheese sandwich with 2 slices of whole wheat bread
1 1/2 ounces of low-fat cheese with 1 teaspoon low-fat mayonnaise
1 medium apple

Snack:
1 medium orange

Supper:
POT ROAST (page 163)
1 WHOLE WHEAT ROLL (page 207)
PEACH COBBLER (page 215)

Snack:
2 cups popcorn air-popped without margarine

Table 17: Analysis of Sample Daily Food Intake

	Break-fast	Lunch	Dinner	Snacks	Actual Servings	Recom-mended Servings
Fruits	1	1	1	1	4	2-4
Vege-tables		1	3		3	3-5
Bread/ Cereal	2	2	1	1	6	6-11
Meat	1		1		2	2-3
Dairy	1	1			2	2-3
Fats	1	1	1 1/2		3 1/2	3-6
Sweets/ Alcohol			1		1	Moderate

Try this analysis using the foods that you ate yesterday. A form to record and analyze your dietary intake is provided on the next page.

Table 18: Analysis of Your Daily Food Intake

	Break-fast	Lunch	Dinner	Snacks	Actual Servings	Recom-mended Servings
Fruits						2-4
Vege-tables						3-5
Breads/ Cereals						6-11
Meat						2-3
Dairy						2-3
Fats						3-6
Sweets/ Alcohol						Moderate

Maintain a Healthy Weight

Maintaining healthy body weight is one of the most important things you can do for your arthritis and to prevent chronic diseases such as hypertension and heart disease. Extra weight can increase pain and joint symptoms. Therefore, achievement of a healthy body weight is a reasonable goal in the treatment of all individuals with arthritis. The maintenance of a healthy body weight is especially important for people with gout, a type of crystalline arthritis and in people with replacement (mechanical) joints.

As a rule of thumb, you can **calculate your healthy body weight** by estimating 100 pounds for the first 5 feet of height and an additional 5 pounds for each inch in women. In men, estimate 106 pounds for the first 5 feet of height and add an additional 6 pounds for each additional inch. The weight for your frame size will be within 10 percent above or below this number.

If you find that you are above a healthy body weight, it is important to change your eating habits. Cut back on portion sizes and decrease your consumption of sweets and high-fat foods. Eating 6 servings of breads and cereals, 2 servings of fruits, 3 servings of vegetables, 2 servings of dairy, and 4-6 ounces of meat a day will provide you with approximately 1200 calories.

Total fasting, the use of very low calorie diets, and fad diets should be avoided. The advice of a physician trained in nutrition or a registered/licensed dietitian can be helpful in weight loss.

Table 19: High-sugar/high-fat foods to limit for weight loss

Margarine/butter	Regular cheese
Candy bars	Pies
Sodas	Candy
Cakes	Ice cream
Cookies	Nuts
Chips	Salad dressings

Choose a Diet Low in Total Fat, Saturated Fat and Cholesterol

It is also important to be aware of how much fat, saturated fat, and cholesterol you are consuming. To be able to include a variety of foods in the diet without exceeding calorie needs, it is necessary to follow a low-fat diet. Fat contains more than twice as many calories as carbohydrates or protein, thus contributing significantly to calorie intake when eaten in large amounts. A high-fat diet is linked to obesity, heart disease, and cancer. A diet low in fat, saturated fat, and cholesterol can help maintain a desirable level of blood cholesterol. As blood cholesterol increases above the desired level (200 mg/dl) there is a greater risk for heart disease. It is recommended that total fat intake should not exceed 30% of total calories and 10% or less should come from saturated fat.

The following table shows foods high in saturated fat. They should be avoided and lower-fat items substituted, when possible.

Table 20: Foods High in Saturated Fat

Butter	Bacon drippings
Lard	Vegetable shortening
Coconut oil	Palm kernel oil
Palm oil margarine	Cocoa butter
Cream	Hardened fat or oils
Animal fat	Poultry skin
Cheese	Whole milk
Chocolate	Sausage and most processed luncheon meats

Suggestions for a Diet Low in Fat, Saturated Fat and Cholesterol

Fats and oil

❑ Do not fry foods.

❑ Use fats and oils sparingly.

- Use small amounts of salad dressings and spreads, margarine and regular mayonnaise.

- Use liquid vegetable oils when possible, but use them sparingly.

- Check labels on foods for fat and saturated fat content.

Meat, poultry, fish, dry beans, and eggs

- Two or three servings, with a daily total not exceeding 6 ounces.

- Three ounces of cooked lean meat or poultry is about the size of a deck of cards.

- Trim fat from meat; remove skin from poultry.

- Have meatless main dishes featuring cooked dry beans and peas.

- Use egg yolks and organ meats in moderate amounts. (limit to 4 egg yolks/week)

Milk and milk products

- Have two or three servings daily (1 cup of low-fat milk or low-fat yogurt or about 1 ounce of cheese counts as a serving).

- Choose skim or low-fat milk and fat-free or low-fat yogurt and cheese.

Choose a Diet With Plenty of Vegetables, Fruits, and Grain Products

By consuming a diet with plenty of whole grain breads and cereals and fruits and vegetables, it is possible to increase the fiber intake of your diet. As a general guide, it is suggested that 20-35 grams of total fiber be consumed per day. **Insoluble fiber** is found in the skins of fruits and vegetables in grains and cereals. Insoluble fiber helps increase bulk in the diet and aids in preventing constipation. **Soluble fiber** is found in fruits and vegetables, oats, barley bran, and dried beans and peas. Including fiber in the diet is helpful in treating or preventing obesity, diabetes, heart disease and cancer. The inclusion of soluble fiber in the diet may be beneficial for lowering your serum cholesterol level. While decreasing the total amount of fat, saturated fat, and cholesterol in the diet, it also is important to increase the amount of fiber in the diet. This can be done by choosing a diet with plenty of vegetables, fruits and grain products. High fiber foods help reduce symptoms of chronic constipation, diverticular disease, and hemorrhoids. A diet that does not include enough fiber may be linked to increased risk for heart disease, cancer and obesity.

Some of the benefits of fiber may be from the food that provides fiber, not from fiber alone. Therefore, it is important to get fiber from foods rather than supplements. Excessive use of fiber supplements can result in malabsorption of some minerals.

The Fiber Pyramid

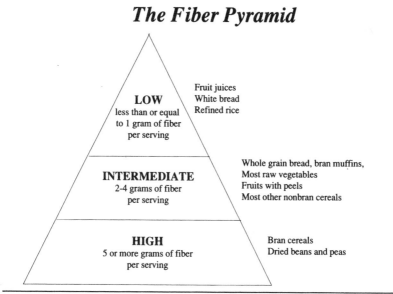

Source: Sarah Morgan, MD, RD, FACP

Very roughly, foods can be stratified into high, intermediate, and low fiber foods. It is recommended that Americans consume 20-35 grams of fiber per day. This pyramid divides food products into the above classifications.

For example, 1 ounce of bran cereal, 2 slices of whole grain bread, 1/2 cup peas, 1/2 cup of baked beans and 1 unpeeled apple = at least 25 grams of fiber.

Use Sugar Only In Moderation

Using sugar in moderation is suggested. Foods which contain large amounts of sugar such as candies, cookies, and desserts are limited in vitamins and minerals. Sugars can also contribute to tooth decay. In addition, labels may not use the word sugar. The following table lists other words for sugar.

Table 21: Different Types of Sugars

Sorbitol	Mannitol	Table sugar (sucrose)
Brown sugar	Molasses	Fruit juice concentrate
Raw sugar	Corn sweetener	Fructose
Corn syrup	Maltose	Honey
Lactose	Dextrose	Glucose

Use Salt and Sodium in Moderation

Salt and sodium should be used in moderation. The Surgeon General suggests 1100 mg - 3300 mg of sodium be consumed per day. One teaspoon of salt contains 2300 mg of sodium. Therefore, one teaspoon of salt contains the total amount of sodium (both added to foods and the sodium in foods) that should be consumed on a daily basis. Removing the salt shaker from the table is one of the easiest ways to lower your intake. Most Americans exceed their sodium needs. A diet high in salt and sodium is associated with high blood pressure, which can lead to heart disease, stroke and kidney disease.

To Moderate the Use of Salt and Sodium

❑ Use salt and flavored salts sparingly in cooking, and avoid use at the table.

❑ Use fresh and frozen vegetables and no-salt-added tomato products.

❑ Cook cereals, pasta, and rice without adding salt. Ready-to-eat cereals are relatively high in sodium.

- All cheeses are high in sodium. Use regular cheese sparingly or look for packages marked "reduced-sodium" or "low-sodium."

- Use fresh meat, poultry, and fish because they are lower in sodium than canned, smoked and processed ones.

- Most frozen dinners and combination dishes, packaged mixes, canned soups, bottled sauces and salad dressings contain a lot of sodium.

- Condiments such as pickles, olives, mustard, Worcestershire sauce, catsup, and soy sauce are very high in sodium. Use low-sodium counterparts when possible.

- Look for unsalted crackers, chips and nuts.

- Check labels for the amount of sodium in foods. Choose those foods that are low-sodium (140 milligrams of sodium or less per serving).

Drink Alcohol In Moderation

Finally, drink alcoholic beverages in moderation or not at all. The definition of moderation is 1-2 drinks a day. One drink is 12 ounces of regular beer, 5 ounces of wine or 1 1/2 ounces of 80 proof liquor. No alcohol should be consumed during pregnancy. Alcoholic beverages supply substantial calories with little or no nutrients. Many arthritis medications including methotrexate, nonsteroidal anti-inflammatory drugs, and colchicine, as well as over the counter drugs including aspirin should not be used with alcohol. Alcohol may reduce the benefits or increase the risk of toxicities with these medications. Drinking alcohol increases the amount of uric acid in the blood, which can further aggravate gouty arthritis. You should consult your physician or pharmacist to determine if alcohol is specifically harmful for your medical condition or interacts with your medication.

Recommended Low-Fat Cookbooks

BE HEART SMART . . . THE HCF WAY TO A HEALTHY HEART by James W. Anderson. HCF Nutrition Research Foundation, 1989.

BEYOND CHOLESTEROL by Peter Kwiterovich. The Johns Hopkins UP, 1989.

CONTROLLING CHOLESTEROL by Kenneth H. Cooper. Bantam Books, 1988.

COOKING ALA HEART by Linda Hachfeld and Betsy Eykyn. Appletree Press, 1992.

COOKING LIGHT COOKBOOK SERIES. Oxmoor House, 1991-1995.

COUNT OUT CHOLESTEROL COOKBOOK: A FEELING FINE BOOK edited by Art Ulene. A. A. Knopf, 1989.

DELICIOUS WAYS TO LOWER CHOLESTEROL by Nedra Wilson and Susan M. Wood. Oxmoor House, 1989.

EATER'S CHOICE: A FOOD LOVER'S GUIDE TO LOWER CHOLESTEROL by Ron Goor and Nancy Goor. Houghton Mifflin, 1989.

FAT AND CHOLESTEROL COUNTER by the American Heart Association. Time Books/Random House, 1991.

GOOD FAT, BAD FAT: HOW TO LOWER YOUR CHOLESTEROL AND BEAT THE ODDS OF A HEART ATTACK by Glen C. Friffen and William P. Castelli. Fisher Books, 1989.

THE JOHNS HOPKINS COMPLETE GUIDE FOR PREVENTING AND REVERSING HEART DISEASE by Peter Kwiterovich and the Lipid Research Clinic Staff. Prima Publishing, 1992.

LOW CHOLESTEROL CUISINE by Anne Lindsay. Morrow, 1992.

LOW-FAT, LOW-CHOLESTEROL COOKBOOK by The American Heart Association. Random House, 1989.

SKIMMING THE FAT: A PRACTICAL FOOD GUIDE by Maureen Callahan. The American Dietetic Association, 1992, item number 0810.

WHAT'S FOR BREAKFAST? LIGHT & EASY MORNING MEALS FOR BUSY PEOPLE by Donna Roy and Kathleen Flores. Appletree Press, 1994.

Chapter 3:
Kitchen
Basics

Contents

Chapter 3
KITCHEN BASICS

Preparing a meal involves much more than cooking. There are menus to be planned, groceries to be bought and stored, ingredients to be mixed, cookware to be selected, and finally dishes to be washed. No wonder people make remarks like:

"Cooking makes me so tired that I don't even want to eat."

"I would do more cooking, but my hands hurt so much."

"Carrying those heavy grocery bags takes all the energy I've got."

There are several reasons why having arthritis makes you feel tired. The first reason is that arthritis causes inflammation around the joints. It takes energy for the body to combat this inflammation — energy which the body gets from food. When your arthritis "flares up", your body uses its natural energy to fight the pain and inflammation. This leaves you with less energy for activities like shopping and cooking. The pain and discomfort of arthritis also causes stress. You may feel that you have to protect your joints to keep them from hurting. You may even have trouble getting a good night's sleep. Stress and sleeplessness "gang-up" on you to rob you of your natural energy in a negative cycle. You are tense because you can't rest, and you can't rest because you are tense.

In some cases, arthritis can change the shape of the joints in the arms and hands. Healthy joints and tendons are designed to make efficient use of the energy stored in muscles. If joints are swollen or damaged, tendons slip to the side, changing their angle of pull. When this happens and hands become stiff, they are less able to grasp and hold. As strength in the hands decreases, additional damage to tendons and joints may occur. In arthritis, inflammation, pain, stress and joint stiffness are all energy-robbers. But there are many ways to outsmart them by using your energy wisely. The secret lies in understanding your disease process and in changing some of your daily habits.

Fighting Back Against Energy-Robbers

Each of the next three sections of this chapter presents ideas to help you simplify meal preparation and save energy. Section 1 discusses the need for an energy-savings plan. Section 2 gives practical advice about making cooking more relaxing. Finally, Section 3 provides additional information about habits and kitchen tools to pamper and protect your joints. Following the tips suggested in this chapter will make preparing and serving nourishing meals easier and more enjoyable.

Section 1: Developing an Energy-Savings Plan

Your body's main energy source is the food you eat every day. Think of food-energy as a deposit into a daily savings account. To manage arthritis, you will want to budget this energy wisely. Using this energy constantly will deplete your energy balance. Regular rest periods and relaxation increase the balance. There are two ways to keep your "energy savings balance" healthy. First you must stop doing things in ways that waste energy. Next, you must make wise choices with the energy you do have. Here are proven ways to end each day with a positive balance in your energy savings account.

Avoid habits which lower your energy balance. Enhance your energy by following these suggestions:

*   Do not work from a standing position. Always sit in a chair with a firm seat and a fairly straight back which supports your back. Rest your arms on a table or counter.

Figure 1 illustrates the best sitting posture.

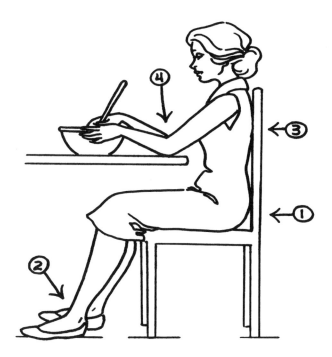

Figure 1

Notice the key points of body support.

    1. Buttocks squarely on the chair.
    2. Both feet on the floor.
    3. Back supported by the chair.
    4. Upper arms relaxed and supported by the table.
    5. Forearms and hands free.

* If you must stand while working, avoid bending over while you are standing.

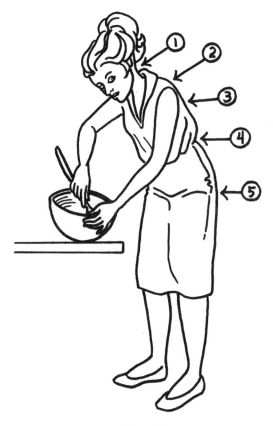

Figure 2

Notice all of the tension points in Figure 2 caused by bending.

      1. Neck
      2. Shoulders
      3. Upper spine
      4. Mid-back
      5. Hips

*   Be sure that your work surface is the correct height.

Work surfaces should be two inches below the elbows when your shoulders are relaxed. If the surface in your work area is too low, you will be wasting valuable energy.

*   Monitor your level of fatigue.

Working when you are already tired is like stealing from your energy savings account. Simplify cooking tasks into several steps, and do only as much at one time as you can without tiring. Try not to begin an activity unless it can be safely interrupted.

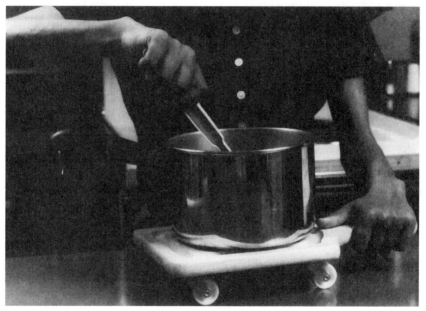

Figure 3

*   Minimize the amount of lifting you do.

Lifting takes lots of energy and can quickly reduce your energy balance. Ask others to help you do things like carrying and storing groceries or mopping the floor. If this is not possible, place heavy objects on a cart with wheels or on rollers.

In addition, adopt kitchen habits which add to your energy balance. There are many things that you can do to keep your energy balance high.

* Rest **before** you get tired. Plan to take short, frequent rest periods throughout the day. Determine the amount of rest your body needs to avoid fatigue.

* Alternate heavy and light, long and short household tasks to avoid working non-stop. Stopping to rest before getting the task completed is desirable and more efficient.

* Organize your workspace. Keep frequently used ingredients and implements between hip and eye level to minimize bending and wasting energy in needless searching. Utilize turntables and pullout shelves in storage areas. A Lazy-Susan can help place ingredients within reach. Keep cleaning supplies together near the area where you will use them. Store ingredients and supplies in small containers to reduce fatigue.

* Adjust to a new attitude that countertops are there to serve you and do not need to be free of useful items. Heavier, more often-used items should be left out on the countertop.

* Shop for pre-cut or pre-packaged food. Convenience foods decrease the amount of time and number of steps in preparing meals, thus reducing fatigue.

* Use labor- and time-saving devices such as an electric skillet, food processor, electric can opener and microwave to enhance your energy balance.

* When cooking, make enough to store, freeze and re-heat for days when you do not feel up to it.

* Use lighter-weight pots, pans and dishes. This will reduce joint stress and fatigue. Avoid heavy stoneware, iron skillets and heavy glass baking dishes.

*   Serve meals buffet-style, letting family members select their own plates, silverware and napkins to eliminate added steps and energy in setting the table. Paper plates and plasticware eliminate dishwashing, thus adding to your energy savings balance on trying days.

*   Minimize clean-up. Prepare one-dish meals that can be served in the same container in which they were cooked. Line pans with foil or use disposable containers to save time and energy. Use a sponge instead of a dishrag to clean surfaces. A sponge can be pressed down with the palm of the hand instead of being wrung to release water.

*   Turn appliances on or off with electric or built-in timers. Select appliances with levers or push buttons, and avoid knobs that are hard to turn. If you are using an external timer, be sure that it has adequate wattage.

*   Ask for help when you are having a bad day. Workloads need to be shared. (Remember that the goal is to end with a positive energy balance each day and reduce the amount of time or need for recovery periods.)

*   Take advantage of the "Quick and Easy" recipes in **THE ESSENTIAL ARTHRITIS COOKBOOK**. They require short preparation time and little effort and are marked with this symbol.

Some days are busier than others. A physician's appointment can fill up your afternoon, or you may have evening dinner plans. It may be your turn to carpool or the day to do the laundry. Whatever the reason, you can plan ahead for these days by choosing a "Quick and Easy" menu. These meals were designed especially for difficult days.

Section 2: Alternate Work Time with Relaxation Time.

It is hard to manage arthritis from day to day without scheduling time to relax. The goal of true relaxation is to remove the tension from the body and tap into natural energy sources. Many of us think of relaxation as "doing nothing." But, **WHEN YOU ARE REALLY RELAXING, YOU ARE DOING SOMETHING IMPORTANT**. You are choosing to pay attention to all the messages your body is giving you. People who know how to relax use four kinds of relaxation activities — mini-breaks, stretch-breaks, relaxation breaks, and rest periods — identified by   in the recipes.

MINI-BREAKS last 1-2 minutes. Use this time to take a deep breath and to locate tension building up in your body. Close your eyes and actively relax these body parts. You need to take a mini-break every ten minutes while you are working.

STRETCH BREAKS last 2-5 minutes. Use this time to change your body's position. Raise your arms and lower them. Get up and walk a little. Take some deep breaths. Shake out the kinks. You need to take a stretch break every twenty minutes while you are working.

RELAXATION PERIODS last fifteen minutes or more. During a relaxation period you should stop working entirely and concentrate solely on relaxation. Take the phone off the hook. Try to clear your mind. Some people find it helpful to use relaxation exercises or guided imagery. If you feel that these techniques might help you, ask your physician or therapist. It is wise to take at least two relaxation breaks a day.

REST PERIODS last over an hour. During a rest break you may want to sit in a comfortable chair or even lie down. The number of rest breaks you need will vary depending on how you feel.

Below is a sample schedule showing how relaxation periods can fit in while you are preparing a meal. Use a kitchen timer to remind you of this pattern of timing yourself to use and restore your energy.

Table 22: Sample Meal Preparation with Relaxation Breaks

Recipe: SKILLET CHICKEN AND VEGETABLES

2	teaspoons olive oil
1	pound boneless and skinless chicken breasts
1	pound small new potatoes, scrubbed
1	10-ounce package of frozen sugar snap peas
1/2	cup water
1/2	teaspoon chicken-flavored bouillon
2	tablespoons dried minced onion

1/4 teaspoon garlic powder
1/2 teaspoon lemon pepper seasoning

Heat olive oil in a large skillet over medium heat; add chicken, and cook until lightly brown, turning as needed. Place vegetables around chicken. Add all other ingredients. Cover and bring to a boil over medium heat; reduce heat and simmer 25 minutes or until potatoes and chicken are tender.

Preparation: WORK STEPS

Measure olive oil.
Unwrap and rinse chicken breasts and set into skillet.
Select new potatoes.

Take a mini-break to notice tension.

Scrub new potatoes at the sink (see Figure 13).
Cut open package of sugar snap peas.

Take a 2-minute sitting "breather."

Turn stove burner to medium heat.
Slide skillet onto burner.
Begin browning chicken lightly.

Take a mini-break to move about while measuring dry ingredients.

Return to stove to continue browning chicken.
When meat is brown, slide skillet off burner.

Take a 2-minute sitting break and stretch.

Measure water and add to skillet.
Place other ingredients into skillet.
Cover and begin cooking.

Take a 20-minute relaxation break while this dish is cooking.

By selecting a one-pot meal like this one, you can afford time to relax.

Section 3: Pamper and Protect your Joints

Managing arthritis also involves protecting painful joints. Joints should be protected from forces which may damage them. It is important to rest your hands when the joints are painful and swollen. But even when your hands don't hurt they still need protection. Here are some things you can do to take care of your hands. In order to respect the sources of pain, it may help for you to learn some basic principles about what happens to your tendons and joints while your hands work. The hand can be described as a bunch of sticks (bones) loosely joined to each other with elastic bands (tendons) and covered by flesh and skin. When the hand is relaxed, the fingers tend to curl in slightly. Make a fist by curling your fingers into your palm as far as pain will allow.

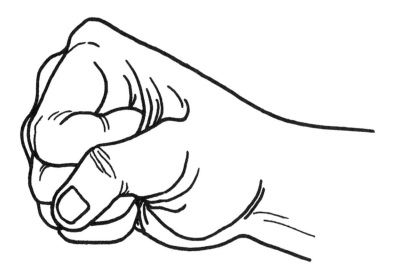

Figure 4

Look at your hand in this position. Notice how the skin is stretched tight over the knuckles. You can see your tendons passing over each joint. In this position, your joints are experiencing the greatest amount of tension. Because of the force and angle of pull, closing your fingers in a tight fist is hard work. Now open your hand and bend your fingers so that they form the letter "C." The tips of your fingers should be 2-3 inches away from the palm, and your thumb should be extended.

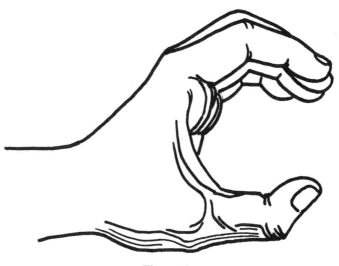

Figure 5

Look at the skin and joints of your hand. The skin is more flexible and the joints look more relaxed. The tendons can slide more easily over the joints. In this position, pain is less likely to occur (Ways of Drawing Hands).

It stands to reason, then, that hands which work in a position resembling a "C" are more relaxed and less prone to injury.

The following illustrations show the desirable "C" position performing a variety of kitchen activities.

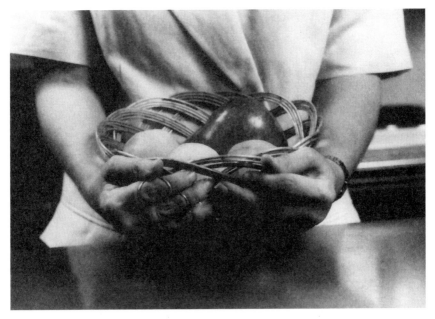

Figure 6

Use the palms of both hands to hold jars or containers, and eliminate tight grasping. Note the use of a lightweight basket.

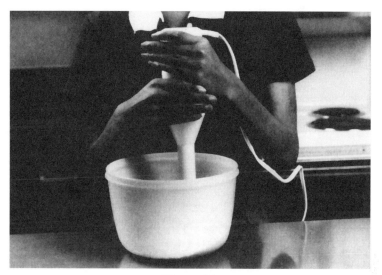

Figure 7A

Use a hand-held mixer to eliminate extra motion.

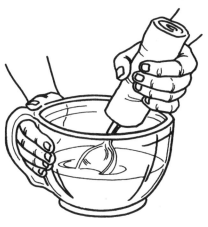

Figure 7B

Build up handles of cutlery by wrapping cloth or foam padding around them to maintain a secure hold.

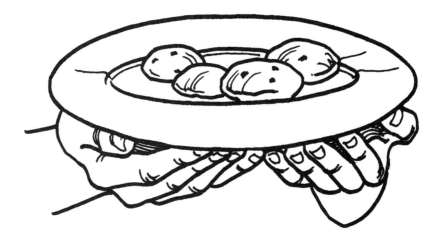

Figure 8

Cup your hands under plates instead of grasping them with your fingertips
to distribute the weight to your palms and avoid joint stress.

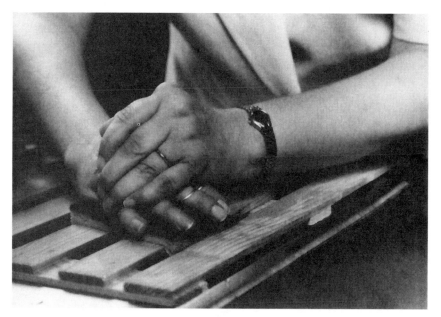

Figure 9

Do not wring out a mop or cloth. Sponge cloths are easier to use and will dry flat or can be pressed dry with a flat hand.

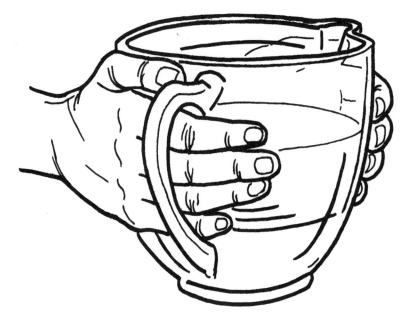

Figure 10

Use lightweight, plastic mixing bowls with big handles so that you can slide your fingers through in the "C" position.

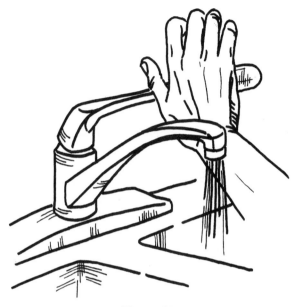

Figure 11

Extend handles on doors or water taps to take advantage of added leverage.

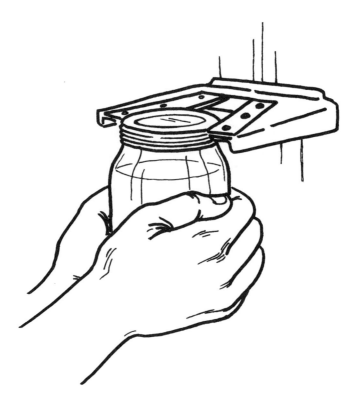

Figure 12

Use a jar opener to loosen lids, while you use both hands to turn the jar.

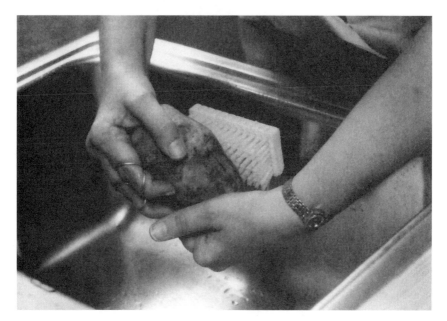

Figure 13

Attach a brush with suction cups in the side of the sink for scrubbing fresh vegetables.

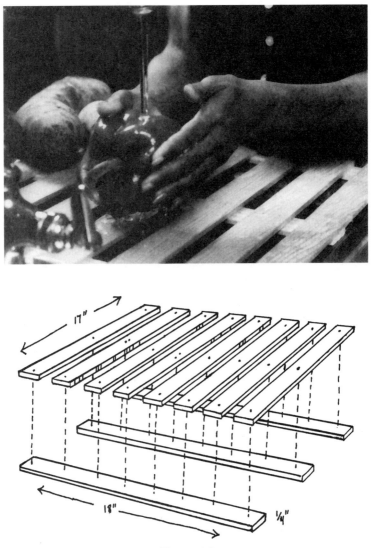

Figure 14

Raise the level of your sink by using a dish-drying rack that fits over the edges. To obtain construction plans for an over-the-counter sink rack, contact: Kitchen Basics, Division of Occupational Therapy, 237 SHRP Building, UAB Station, Birmingham, AL 35294-1270.

Selecting the Right Tools

The weight and shape of the tools you use in the kitchen also affects your joints. Here are other ideas to help protect your hands and prevent joint pain.

* Use light-weight dishes and utensils. Plastic is lighter than crockery, aluminum is lighter than steel, paper is lightest of all. Baskets are also useful.

* Use large-handled kitchen tools. Many types of tools come with large plastic or rubber handles. If you prefer, you can slide foam rubber tubing over the handle to increase the size. Foam rubber tubing is used as pipe insulation and can be purchased at a hardware store.

* Use electric appliances to do the work of your hands. Electric appliances include can openers, electric knives or slicers, mixers, rice cookers, crock pots, salad shooters, food processors and bread makers.

* Boil vegetables or pasta in a pot lined with a mesh basket. Place the mesh basket or food strainer inside the pot before putting food in. When you lift up on the basket, water will drain naturally.

* Use a kitchen scissors to open paper packaging. A lightweight scissors made of plastic or aluminum is a good substitute for a knife. Keep it by your work area for opening cellophane bags and cardboard cartons.

* Use your sink's sprayer hose to fill pots or other containers. Place the empty pot on the counter and not down in the sink. A pot filled in the sink will be too heavy to lift when it is full. Slide the filled pot along the counter onto the burner.

* Wear an apron with pockets. Objects you use frequently (like measuring spoons or scissors) can be stored in the pockets so they will be close by when you need them.

* Become familiar with the housewares section at the store. Many gadgets are available to make cooking easier. For more ideas, see our review of kitchen tools below.

Review of Kitchen Tools

It would be impossible to list every available kitchen tool or gadget. The alphabetical list which follows gives you a good idea of what to choose and what to avoid.

Apple Corer Choose one with a large handle of wood or plastic.

Bulb Baster Small amounts of liquid can be added or removed from a container even when grasp is weak.

Blender A blender or food processor is a must for your kitchen. Be sure to choose one that comes apart easily and whose container and lid are dishwasher safe.

Bottle Opener Avoid caps which must be pried off. Large twist-off caps can be opened with a jar opener.

Bottle Stopper Stoppers made of cork, rubber or soft plastic are useful for recapping open containers. Choose ones with broad flat tops so that you can push them down using the palm of your hand.

Butter Melter Butter or other shortening can be melted in a microwave. Try to melt it in the container in which it will be used.

Canister Put ingredients like flour, rice, or sugar into lightweight canisters. Store canisters on a Lazy-Susan centrally in your work area.

Can Opener/Electric can opener Sponges can be stacked under large cans to support some of the weight. A long handle on the operating lever will increase your leverage.

Casserole Dish These containers are essential for one-pot meals. Keep an assortment of sizes. Avoid metal casseroles which are heavier and cannot be used in a microwave oven.

Cheese Cloth This thin cotton can be used as a strainer and weighs next to nothing.

Chopper A food chopper or a chopping jar allows you to cut food without gripping a knife.

Colander A large colander is useful for holding vegetables while you rinse them with a rubber sprayer. Place a dish drainer over the sink and rest the colander on it.

Cookbook Holder This clear, acrylic holder keeps your cookbook clean from splatters and spills and keeps pages conveniently open.

Cookie Sheet Non-stick, non-burn baking sheets are now available. If you use any other kind, cover the surface with foil or parchment paper for easy clean-up.

Cupcake Liners Use paper inserts not only for baking but also in portioning individual servings of puddings or similar desserts in the refrigerator.

Cutting Board Suction cups under a cutting board will keep it from shifting on the work surface. Two aluminum nails, placed one inch apart and protruding from the cutting surface can be used to stabilize meat and vegetables. Plastic wrap placed over the board and extending 3-4 inches on all sides will minimize clean-up.

Dish Drainer A dish drainer which fits over the sink will let you work at the level of your counter. A simple pattern for construction of a wooden drainer is illustrated in Figure 14 of this book.

Egg Slicer This gadget slices hard boiled eggs using thin wires. It can also give good leverage for cutting other soft ingredients like butter.

Flour Sifter Today's flour needs little sifting. If you must use a sifter, avoid the one which you squeeze. Sift only small amounts at a time.

Fruit Juicer Even an electric juicer uses a lot of your energy. You would be better to buy juice at the store.

Garlic Press This is an energy-robber. Chopped garlic is commercially available.

Grater Yet another energy-robber. Use a food processor for vegetables, fruits or cheese. Buy pre-ground spices such as nutmeg, cinnamon, cloves or orange zest.

Kettle If you use a kettle frequently, consider using a "kettle-tipper" which allows you to pour without lifting.

Kitchen Shears Trim fats from meat using shears. Be sure to select a pair that can be washed in the dishwasher.

Kitchen Stool A high stool with a back and foot rest will let you sit while you work at the sink. Be sure that you choose one with a stable base of support. Rubber tips on the feet will keep the stool from sliding on the floor.

Ladle A one-cup measurement or less allows you to serve chili, soup and stew without lifting the entire pot.

Lazy-Susan This circular, rotating tray puts things within reach. You may want to use several — one for spices, one for staples, and one to keep frequently-used utensils at your fingertips.

Mixing Bowl A damp paper towel placed on the work surface will keep the bowl from turning. Unbreakable plastic bowls are lighter and are safe for the dishwasher. Bowls with handles are easier to stabilize during use even if they are more difficult to store.

Measuring Cup Choose plastic over glass. Be sure to use one which you can see through, as it makes exact measuring easier.

Measuring Spoons Plastic or aluminum will do. Store an extra set of measuring spoons inside canisters of ingredients you use frequently such as sugar and flour.

Pancake Turner These are useful for turning any food which you cook in a pan. Plastic is lighter, but may tend to melt in high heat. Be sure to choose one with a large handle.

Potato Peeler This may be substituted for a vegetable peeler and usually comes with a larger handle.

Pot Holder Use plenty of these. They not only protect you from heat but can be wrapped around handles to build them up. The thicker the better. Mitt potholders allow you to lift and hold casserole bowls with the palms of both hands.

Rubber Handles Various sizes of foam rubber tubing are available at most hardware stores. Using foam tubing on kitchen tools increases the size of the handles and makes them non-slip.

Salad Basket These small wire baskets are good for rinsing any fresh vegetable or any dried foods such as beans.

Scraper Rubber spatulas are useful for transferring dough or other mixtures from one container to another. Some rubber spatulas are shaped like a shallow spoon.

Slotted Spoon These are useful for many different cooking tasks. Remember to choose by weight and handle size.

Soft-drink openers A long flat piece of metal, similar to a letter opener, can be placed under tabs for opening.

Timer Set timers for cooking but also use them to signal the beginning or end of a relaxation period.

Tongs There are several types of tongs on the market. They are useful for serving food and for turning meats or vegetables. Thin-handled tongs can be built-up using a pot holder.

Warming Tray Trays are especially useful when family members eat at different times. Most have a "hot spot" to keep food warm.

Wire Whisk Although useful for whipping ingredients, the slim handle generally makes this a poor choice.

Wheeled Trivet A small, wheeled platform placed under a heavy appliance (such as a crock pot or blender) can eliminate lifting.

Vegetable Peeler The double edge of a vegetable peeler is useful for scraping carrots or potatoes. Look for the style that fits over the fingers. Its shape does not require a strong grip.

User-Friendly Kitchen Tools

There are many special products on the market including the following:

Cookbook holders	Rolling trivets
Door knob extensions	Non-skid pads
Extended drinking straws	E-Z grip knives
Over-the-sink cutting boards	Pan holders
Jar lid openers	Handles for milk cartons

Suppliers for these specialty items include the following:

AdaptAbility
P.O. Box 51
Colchester, CT 06415-0515
1-800-243-9232
(products for independent living)

Cleo of New York
Trent Building
S. Buckout Street
Irvington, NY 10533
1-800-431-2830

Enrichments
#4 Sammons Court
Bolingbrook, IL 60440
1-800-323-5547

Sammons
#4 Sammons Court
Bolingbrook, IL 60440
1-800-323-5547
(adaptive tableware, hand/wrist cuffs, food
guards, scooper plates)

Appletree Press Inc.
Suite 125
151 Good Counsel Drive
Mankato, MN 56001
1-800-322-5679
(cookbook holders, kitchen tools)

Aids for Arthritis Inc.
3 Little Knoll Court
Medford, NJ 08055
609-654-6918
(jar openers, grippers, videos, non-slip mixing bowls)

American Able Data
1-800-364-2742
Provides information on where to get specially adapted tools from the National Rehabilitative Data Service.

Be sure to read the product descriptions and specifications in the catalog before you purchase. Even the handiest gadget is no bargain if left unused.

Resources

A WORKBOOK FOR PERSONS WITH RHEUMATOID ARTHRITIS, by G. Furst, L. H. Gerber, L.H. and C. Smith. U.S. Department of Health and Human Services: 1985. This book is available from the authors by writing Gloria Furst, OTR. National Institutes of Health, Rehabilitation Medicine Department, Building 10, Room 6S235 9000 Rockville Pike, Bethesda, MD 20892.

WAYS OF DRAWING HANDS, Copyright © by Inklink 1994. Published by Running Press Book Publishers.

MEALTIME MANUAL FOR PEOPLE WITH DISABILITIES AND AGING, by J. L. Klinger. Institute of Rehabilitation, New York University Medical Center, and Campbell Soup Company, 1978.

THE ARTHRITIS HELP BOOK, by K. Lorig and J. Fries. Reading: Addison-Wesley Publishing Company, 1986.

Chapter 4:
Menu
Planning

Contents

Chapter 4
MENU PLANNING

A healthy meal plan includes a variety of food each day from the Food Guide Pyramid (see *Chapter 2* for more information).

> 6-11 servings from the bread/grain group
> 3-5 servings of vegetables
> 2-4 servings of fruits
> 2-3 servings of low-fat dairy foods
> 2-3 servings of lean meats, fish, legumes, eggs

What is a Serving?

Breads, Cereals, Rice, & Pasta Group
1 slice bread
1/2 cup cooked rice or pasta
1/2 cup cooked cereal
1 ounce ready-to-eat cereal

Fruit Group
1 piece fruit or melon wedge
3/4 cup juice
1/2 cup canned fruit
1/4 cup dried fruit

Milk, Yogurt, & Cheese Group
1 cup milk or yogurt
1 1/2 ounces natural cheese
2 ounces processed cheese

Vegetable Group
1/2 cup chopped raw or
   cooked vegetables
1 cup leafy raw vegetables

Meat, Poultry, Fish, Dry Beans, Eggs, & Nuts Group
2 1/2 - 3 oz cooked lean meat,
   poultry, or fish (count 1/2
   cup cooked beans or 1 egg
   or 2 tablespoons peanut
   butter as 1 ounce of lean
   meat)

Fats, Oils, & Sweets
1 teaspoon margarine
2 tablespoons fat-free salad
   dressing
1 small slice cake
1-2 small cookies
   or 1 medium cookie

Ways to Reach These Goals

❑ You will usually need bread at each meal to get 6-11 servings from that group, even though most meals will include pasta, rice or a grain food.

❑ Soup or salad and bread help complete one-dish meals or meals built around frozen dinners.

❑ Choose low-fat milk to complement your meals or snacks.

❑ Fresh fruits are delightful for dessert.

❑ Raw vegetables make easy, portable snacks.

Important Components of Meal Planning

❑ Taste

❑ Appearance

❑ Texture

❑ Temperature

In addition, people with arthritis, fibromyalgia and other chronic pain and fatigue need to consider:

❑ Time

❑ Energy

Minimizing time and energy in meal preparation by effective meal planning reduces stress on joints and lessens pain.

A Week of Sample Menus

DAY 1

Breakfast   Bran Flakes Cereal
Skim Milk
Whole, Fresh Strawberries

Lunch   Tuna Sandwich: Whole Wheat Bread
Tuna, packed in water
Reduced-Fat Mayonnaise
Pickle Relish
Lettuce Leaf
Tomato Slices
Raw Cauliflower
Fat-Free Ranch Dressing
Kiwi Fruit

Dinner   ROASTED PORK LOIN (page 167)
SPICED SWEET POTATOES WITH
  APPLES (page 180)
LEMON-PEPPER SPINACH (page 176)
Dinner Roll
Fat-Free Ice Cream topped with Cherry Preserves
Tea

Approximate Total Calories Per Day: 1359
Approximate Calories From Fat: 19%

DAY 2

Breakfast   Fruited Yogurt Topped with Low-fat Granola
DROP BISCUITS (page 206)
Margarine
Coffee

Lunch   Roasted Turkey Sandwich
  with Chopped Fresh Vegetables
  in Pita Pocket with Mustard
Orange Slices
Skim Milk

Dinner	Zucchini Lasagna (frozen dinner)
	French Bread
	Tossed Salad (pre-packaged)
	Fat-free Italian Dressing
	SPICY FRUIT BAKE (page 229)
	Water with Lemon Wedge

Approximate Total Calories Per Day: 1305
Approximate Calories From Fat: 19%

DAY 3

Breakfast	Oatmeal
	Toasted BATTER BREAD (page 192)
	Orange Juice
	Skim Milk

Lunch	POTATO SOUP (page 111)
	Chopped Cucumbers, Tomatoes and
	Onions in vinegar
	Cheese Toast
	Grapes
	Tea

Dinner	SKILLET CHICKEN AND VEGETABLES (page 156
	French Roll
	CHEWY DATE SQUARES (page 222)
	Iced Tea

Approximate Total Calories Per Day: 1290
Approximate Calories From Fat: 20%

DAY 4

Breakfast	RAISIN BRAN MUFFIN (page 203)
	Melon Wedge
	Skim Milk

Lunch	BROCCOLI-TOPPED POTATO (page 134)

	Whole Grain Bread
	Sliced Tomatoes
	Peach
	Skim Milk

Dinner	Glazed Chicken on Rice
	with French Green Beans (frozen dinner)
	MANDARIN ORANGE SALAD (page 120)
	Dinner Roll
	Tea

Approximate Total Calories Per Day: 1339
Approximate Calories From Fat: 13%

DAY 5

Breakfast	Grapefruit Half
	Boiled Egg
	Toasted English Muffin
	Margarine
	Skim Milk

On-the-Run Lunch	Fast-Food Single Hamburger
	with Catsup, Mustard, Pickle
	Green Side Salad with Light Vinaigrette
	Small Yogurt Cone
	Orange Juice

Dinner	BAKED ORANGE ROUGHY (page 142)
	BLACK-EYED PEAS AND RICE (page 185)
	Steamed Cabbage
	Dinner Roll
	RAISIN BREAD PUDDING (page 232)
	with VANILLA CUSTARD SAUCE (page 211)
	Coffee

Approximate Total Calories Per Day: 1643
Approximate Calories From Fat: 19%

DAY 6

Breakfast   BANANA, ORANGE, PINEAPPLE
          BEVERAGE (page 94)
          Bagel with Fat-Free Cream Cheese

Lunch   BEEF STEW (page 157)
          Saltine Crackers
          Pear
          Skim Milk

Dinner   BROCCOLI RICE CASSEROLE (page 133)
          Tomato Aspic (canned)
          Dinner Roll
          Baked Apple
          Hot Tea with Lemon

Approximate Total Calories Per Day: 1346
Approximate Calories From Fat: 14%

DAY 7

Breakfast   POTATO CHEESE FRITTATA (page 135)
          BANANA NUT BREAD (page 191)
          Grapefruit Juice
          Skim Milk

Lunch   CHICKEN & RICE SALAD on Lettuce
           Leaf (page 148)
          Chilled Asparagus Spears (canned)
          Fresh Pineapple Chunks (pre-packaged)
          Melba Toast
          Peanut Butter Cookie
          Iced Tea

Dinner   TAMALE PIE (page 165)
          Coleslaw with Mayonnaise Dressing (pre-packaged)
          Angel Food Cake
           with Orange Sherbet and Fresh Blueberries

Approximate Total Calories Per Day: 1294
Approximate Calories From Fat: 17%

Additional calories for a more active lifestyle and to prevent weight loss can be provided by nutritious snacks such as:

*   Fruits

*   Cereals

*   Skim milk

*   Breads, crackers

*   Low-fat cheese or lean meat

*   Low-fat cookies and cakes in moderation

Recipes

Contents

A Word About the Recipes

Recipes in THE ESSENTIAL ARTHRITIS COOKBOOK are specially developed to reduce preparation **time**, the **number** of bowls and utensils and the **range of motion** needed in the kitchen. All recipes have been tested by a number of taste-testers and prepared by people with arthritis to certify that they produce tasty dishes time after time with a minimal amount of energy.

 Look for this logo at the top of recipes that are "Quick and Easy."

Mini-rest or stretch breaks are designated by this special figure ☺.
Refer to *Chapter 3* (page 50) for more information on mini-rest and stretch breaks.

All recipes are low in fat and cholesterol, moderate in the amount of salt and sugar, and fit into a well-balanced diet.

Recipes have been analyzed for nutritional value using the Nutrition Data System (NDS) from the University of Minnesota. Nutrition analysis includes total calories, protein, carbohydrate, fat, saturated fat, cholesterol and sodium. The percentage of calories from fat is also given for dishes that are or could be considered as a main entree. Diabetic exchanges are also given.

HEALTHIER SUBSTITUTIONS LIST

Ingredient	Substitution
Bacon	Lean ham
Baking chocolate (1 square)	3 tablespoons cocoa + 1 tablespoon vegetable oil
Bouillon	Reduced-sodium bouillon or broth
Butter/margarine	Reduced by one-third
Cheese	Part-skim milk or reduced-fat cheese
Cottage cheese	Low-fat cottage cheese
Coconut	Dried fruit
Cream	Skim milk
Cream cheese	Light cream cheese, Neufchatel or fat-free cream cheese
Egg	2 egg whites or egg substitute
Evaporated milk	Evaporated skim milk
Fruit packed in syrup	Fruit packed in water or its own juice
Garlic salt	Garlic powder
Ground beef	Ground round
Ground turkey	93% fat-free ground turkey
Ice cream	Fat-free ice cream, low-fat or fat-free frozen yogurt, sherbet or sorbet

Marinades, bottled	Fruit and vegetable juices (like pineapple and tomato)
Mayonnaise	Reduced-calorie or fat-free mayonnaise
Onion salt	Onion powder
Pie crust	Graham cracker or vanilla wafer crumb crust
Salt	Reduce by one-half in recipes and use more seasonings
Shortening	Oil or vegetable cooking spray
Soups	Reduced-fat/reduced-sodium soups
Sour cream	Reduced-fat or fat-free sour cream or nonfat plain yogurt
Soy sauce	Reduced-sodium soy sauce
Sugar	Reduce by one-third in recipes
Tuna packed in oil	Tuna packed in water
Whole buttermilk	Skim buttermilk
Whole milk	1% or skim milk
Whole milk cottage cheese	1% or fat-free cottage cheese
Whole milk Ricotta cheese	Skim milk Ricotta cheese
Worcestershire sauce	Reduced-sodium Worcestershire sauce
Yogurt	Low-fat or fat-free yogurt

WEIGHTS AND MEASURES

Dash	less than 1/8 teaspoon
3 teaspoons	1 tablespoon
4 tablespoons	1/4 cup
8 tablespoons	1/2 cup
12 tablespoons	3/4 cup
16 tablespoons	1 cup
2 cups	1 pint
2 pints	1 quart
4 quarts	1 gallon
16 ounces	1 pound
8 fluid ounces	1 cup
1 ounce	2 tablespoons

FOOD EQUIVALENTS

1 ounce cheese	1/4 cup shredded cheese
1 medium apple	1 cup sliced apple
1 medium banana	3/4 cup sliced banana
1 stick margarine	1/2 cup margarine
1 medium onion	1 cup chopped onion
1 pound potatoes	3 medium potatoes
1 pound boneless, skinless chicken	2 1/2 cups chopped, cooked chicken

Use this space to record recipes you've tried from THE ESSENTIAL ARTHRITIS COOKBOOK and want to have available for quick reference.

RECIPE TITLE   PAGE #

Appetizers

Contents

COLD FRUIT SOUP

6 servings

1	6-ounce package diced mixed dried fruit
1/4	cup quick cooking tapioca
1	quart water
1	cup canned tart red cherries
3/4	cup orange juice
1/2	cup sugar
1	stick cinnamon

Mix first three ingredients in a saucepan and let stand 5 minutes.

Add remaining ingredients and bring to a boil over high heat, stirring constantly. Remove from heat and discard the cinnamon stick.

Chill before serving.

Serving size: 1 cup
Analysis per serving: 188 Calories, 1 g Protein, 46 g Carbohydrate,
0 g Fat, 0 g Sat Fat, 0 mg Cholesterol, 7 mg Sodium
Diabetic exchanges: 2 fruits & 1 starch

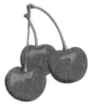

FRUIT & CHEESE SNACK TRAY

6 servings

1	*fresh pear*
1	*fresh apple*
1/2	*pound seedless grapes*
1	*pint strawberries, washed and hulled*
3	*ounces reduced-fat Cheddar cheese*

Wash and cut the pear and apple into 4 pieces each. Core and cut each of these pieces into 3 slices. Cut cheese into 6 slices. Arrange fruit and cheese on a serving tray.

Hint: Dip the apple and pear slices in orange juice immediately after slicing to prevent browning.

Serving size: 1 slice cheese, 1 small cluster of grapes, 2 slices pear, 2 slices apple, and 3 strawberries.
Analysis per serving: 111 Calorie , 5 g Protein, 18 g Carbohydrate, 3 g Fat, 2 g Sat Fat, 0 mg Cholesterol, 76 mg Sodium
Diabetic exchanges: 1 fruit & 1/2 medium-fat meat

ARTICHOKE DIP

1 3/4 cups or 28 servings

1	*14-ounce can artichokes, drained*
1/2	*cup fat-free mayonnaise*
1 1/2	*ounce can grated Parmesan cheese*
84	*pieces Melba Toast*

Chop drained artichokes and place in a medium-sized bowl. Stir in the remaining ingredients and spoon into a small oven-proof bowl.

Heat in a microwave or 350° oven until hot.

Serving size: 1 tablespoon dip evenly spread over 3 pieces of Melba Toast
Analysis per serving: 42 Calories, 1 g Protein, 6 g Carbohydrate,
2 g Fat, 1 g Sat Fat, 1 mg Cholesterol, 142 mg Sodium
Diabetic exchange: 1/2 starch

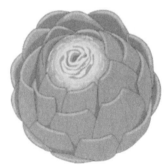

BANANA, ORANGE & PINEAPPLE BEVERAGE

3 servings

1   *cup unsweetened pineapple-orange juice**
1   *8-ounce carton low-fat vanilla yogurt*
2   *medium-sized ripe bananas*

Place all ingredients in a large measuring cup and blend with a hand-held mixer or process in an electric blender, until smooth.

Serve immediately, or cover and refrigerate until ready to serve.

* Plain orange juice can be used in place of pineapple-orange juice.

Serving size: 3/4 cup
Analysis per serving: 193 Calories, 5 g Protein, 45 g Carbohydrate,
1 g Fat, tr Sat Fat, 3 mg Cholesterol, 46 mg Sodium
Diabetic exchanges: 2 1/2 fruits & 1/2 skim milk

CRANBERRY PUNCH

12 servings

4	*cups low-calorie cranberry juice cocktail*
4	*cups unsweetened apple juice*
4	*cups low-calorie lemon-lime soda*

Chill all punch ingredients. When ready to serve, pour juices and soda into punch bowl. Serve immediately.

An ice ring made of additional, low-calorie cranberry juice cocktail will keep your punch chilled while serving.

Serving size: 1 cup
Analysis per serving: 47 Calories, 0 g Protein, 11 g Carbohydrate,
0 g Fat, 0 g Sat Fat, 0 mg Cholesterol, 14 mg Sodium
Diabetic exchange: 1 fruit

SPICED TEA

40 servings

2	*cups orange-flavored breakfast drink with 10% less sugar*
1/2	*cup instant tea with lemon and artificial sweetener*
1	*teaspoon ground cloves*
1	*teaspoon ground cinnamon*

Hot water

Place all ingredients in a jar with a lid or in a reclosable plastic bag. Shake to combine.

Place 1 tablespoon of tea mixture in a cup and add 6 ounces hot water. Stir and serve hot.

Serving size: 1 tablespoon
Analysis per serving: 46 Calories, tr Protein, 11 g Carbohydrate,
tr Fat, 0 g Sat Fat, 0 mg Cholesterol, 1 mg Sodium
Diabetic exchange: 1 fruit

HOLIDAY CHEESE SPREAD

16 servings

1	*8-ounce package fat-free cream cheese*
1	*8-ounce can crushed pineapple in its own juice, drained*
1/4	*cup frozen chopped green pepper*
2	*tablespoons frozen chopped onion*
2	*tablespoons chopped pimento*
1	*teaspoon dried parsley*

Allow cream cheese to soften at room temperature about one hour. Drain pineapple and discard juice.

Combine all ingredients except parsley in a small bowl. Cover and chill. Sprinkle parsley over top of cheese spread before serving.

Serve with fat-free crackers or Melba toast rounds.

Serving size: 2 tablespoons
Analysis per serving: 23 Calories, 2 g Protein, 3 g Carbohydrate,
tr Fat, 0 g Sat Fat, 2 mg Cholesterol, 71 mg Sodium
Diabetic exchange: 1 vegetable

NUTS & BOLTS

18 servings

3	*cups wheat cereal squares*
2	*cups corn cereal squares*
3	*cups rice cereal squares*
1/2	*cup unsalted dry roasted peanuts*
1	*cup pretzels*
1	*tablespoon margarine*
1/4	*teaspoon garlic powder*
1/2	*teaspoon onion powder*
3	*tablespoons low-sodium Worcestershire sauce*
1	*tablespoon lemon juice*

Combine cereals, peanuts, and pretzels in a 13 x 9 x 2 inch baking pan.

Melt margarine in a small saucepan; add remaining ingredients and stir to mix. Pour margarine mixture over cereal mixture, stirring until well coated.

Spread evenly in pan. Bake at 250° for 45 minutes, stirring every 15 minutes. Store in an airtight container, such as a reclosable plastic bag.

Serving size: 1/2 cup
Analysis per serving: 103 Calories, 3 g Protein, 17 g Carbohydrate,
3 g Fat, tr Sat Fat, 0 mg Cholesterol, 183 mg Sodium
Diabetic exchanges: 1 starch & 1/2 fat

Soups

Contents

CHICKEN NOODLE SOUP

One pound of boneless, skinless chicken breast
will yield about 2 1/2 cups of chopped, cooked chicken.
10 servings

1	*pound boneless, skinless chicken breasts*
4	*cups water*
2	*teaspoons chicken-flavored bouillon granules*
1/4	*teaspoon crushed thyme*
1/4	*teaspoon dried chervil*
1/2	*teaspoon salt*
1/4	*teaspoon pepper*
2	*cups egg yolk-free noodles*

Place chicken and water in a Dutch oven. Cover and bring to a boil. Reduce heat and simmer 30 minutes or until tender.

Use a slotted spoon to remove chicken from broth. Chop chicken and return to broth.

Add remaining ingredients and stir to mix. Return to a boil; reduce heat, and simmer for 12 minutes to cook noodles.

Serving size: 2/3 cup
Analysis per serving: 103 Calories, 10 g Protein, 11 g Carbohydrate,
2 g Fat, tr Sat Fat, % Calories from Fat 16, 22 mg Cholesterol, 297 mg Sodium
Diabetic exchanges: 1 starch & 1 lean meat

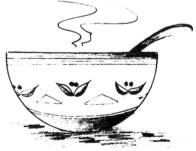

CHICKEN VELVET SOUP

10 servings

1/3	cup reconstituted Butter Buds®
3/4	cup all-purpose flour
6	cups hot chicken broth, divided
2 1/2	cups evaporated skim milk
2	cups diced cooked chicken
1/4	teaspoon salt
1/8	teaspoon pepper

Blend liquid Butter Buds® and flour with a wire whisk in a large nonstick saucepan. Gradually add 2 cups broth, mixing well until smooth.

Add milk, and continue stirring until thickened.

Add remaining chicken broth, chicken, salt and pepper and heat through, stirring as needed to prevent sticking.

Serving size: 1 cup
Analysis per serving: 154 Calories, 16 g Protein, 15 g Carbohydrate,
3 g Fat, 1 g Sat Fat, % Calories from Fat 15, 26 mg Cholesterol, 329 mg Sodium
Diabetic exchanges: 2 lean meats & 1 starch

CREAM OF CHICKEN SOUP

5 servings

1	*pound boneless, skinless chicken breasts*
2	*cups water*
1	*14 1/2-ounce can ready-to-serve chicken broth*
1	*cup evaporated skim milk*
1/2	*cup all-purpose flour*
1/4	*teaspoon crushed thyme*
1/4	*teaspoon dried chervil*
1/2	*teaspoon salt*
1/4	*teaspoon pepper*

Place chicken and water in a saucepan. Cover and bring to a boil. Reduce heat and simmer 30 minutes or until chicken is done. Remove chicken from liquid, reserving liquid.

Mix canned chicken broth and evaporated milk in a small bowl. Add flour and blend with a whisk or hand-held mixer. Add to liquid remaining in saucepan.

Cook over medium heat, stirring constantly, until thickened. Stir in chicken, thyme, chervil, salt, and pepper. Cook over low heat until thoroughly heated.

Serving size: 3/4 cup
Analysis per serving: 145 Calories, 18 g Protein, 11 g Carbohydrate,
2 g Fat, 1 g Sat Fat, % Calories from Fat 12, 39 mg Cholesterol, 497 mg Sodium
Diabetic exchanges: 2 lean meats & 1 starch

SEAFOOD GUMBO

There are many ingredients in a good gumbo, but this recipe is easy and makes enough to freeze. Cook fresh rice to serve with it when reheating. Filé powder can be found in the spice section.

12 servings

1 1/2	*quarts water*
1/2	*pound orange roughy*
1	*pound frozen, peeled, deveined shrimp (uncooked)*
1	*10-ounce box frozen okra*
1	*15-ounce can stewed tomatoes*
1	*cup fresh or frozen chopped onion*
1	*6-ounce can tomato paste*
1/4	*teaspoon ground thyme*
1 1/2	*teaspoons hot sauce*
2	*tablespoons low-sodium Worcestershire sauce*
1/2	*teaspoon pepper*
1 1/2	*teaspoon salt*
1	*tablespoon filé powder*
1/4	*cup flour*
1/2	*cup water*
6	*cups hot cooked rice (cooked without salt or fat)*

Place first 12 ingredients in a nonstick Dutch oven. Cover and bring to a boil. Reduce heat, cover and simmer for 20 minutes or until vegetables are tender, stirring as needed to prevent sticking.☺

Add filé powder to gumbo mixture and stir. In a small bowl, combine the flour and water. Add flour mixture to gumbo mixture and stir. Continue to cook until gumbo thickens.

To serve, place 1/2 cup cooked rice in a bowl and add 1 cup of the gumbo.

Serving size: 1 cup
Analysis per serving: 205 Calories, 14 g Protein, 32 g Carbohydrate,
2 g Fat, tr Sat Fat, % Calories from fat 10, 61 mg Cholesterol, 457 mg Sodium
Diabetic exchanges: 1 1/2 lean meats, 1 1/2 starches & 1 vegetable

BEEF BARLEY SOUP

If quick cooking barley is used, add with vegetables.
Ask your butcher to cut a half pound round steak into cubes.
6 servings

1/2	*pound lean beef, cut for stew*
	Vegetable cooking spray
3 1/2	*cups water*
1	*teaspoon beef-flavored bouillon granules*
1/4	*cup pearl barley*
1/4	*teaspoon salt*
1/4	*teaspoon pepper*
1/2	*teaspoon dried Italian seasoning*
1	*16-ounce package frozen vegetable soup mix with tomatoes*

Cook beef in a Dutch oven coated with cooking spray over medium heat until meat is brown.

Add water, bouillon granules, barley, salt, pepper and Italian seasoning. Cover and bring to a boil; reduce heat and simmer 1 hour, stirring occasionally. ☺

Add vegetables, and continue to cook, covered, 20 minutes or until meat and vegetables are tender.

Serving size: 1 cup
Analysis per serving: 141 Calories, 13 g Protein, 16 g Carbohydrate,
2 g Fat, 1 g Sat Fat, % Calories from fat 13, 28 mg Cholesterol, 339 mg Sodium
Diabetic exchanges: 2 lean meats, 1/2 starch & 1 vegetable

Vegetable Beef Soup

10 servings

1	*pound ground round*
1	*14 1/2-ounce can ready-to-serve beef broth*
1	*16-ounce package of frozen vegetable soup mix with tomatoes*
2	*tablespoons low-sodium Worcestershire sauce*
Dash pepper	
1/4	*teaspoon crushed thyme*
1/4	*teaspoon crushed marjoram*
1	*14 1/2-ounce can Italian stewed tomatoes*
3	*cups water*

Cook meat in Dutch oven over medium heat until meat is brown, stirring to crumble meat. Add all other ingredients and stir to mix. Cover and bring to a boil; reduce heat, and simmer for 45 minutes.

Serving size: 1 cup
Analysis per serving: 118 Calories, 13 g Protein, 10 g Carbohydrate,
3 g Fat, 1 g Sat Fat, % Calories from Fat 21, 33 mg Cholesterol, 434 mg Sodium
Diabetic exchanges: 1 lean meat & 2 vegetables

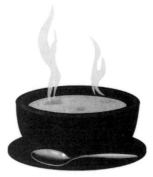

MIXED BEAN SOUP

If you prefer a milder flavor, use plain stewed tomatoes.
A purchased bean soup mix may contain a seasoning packet.
Discard it if the list of ingredients includes salt.
6 servings

1	*cup bean soup mixture*
1	*quart water*
2	*ounces (1/2 cup) lean cubed ham*
1/4	*teaspoon pepper*
8	*ounces (1 cup) stewed tomatoes with green chiles*
1/2	*teaspoon salt*
1/4	*teaspoon dried minced garlic*
1/2	*cup chopped fresh or frozen onion*
2	*tablespoons lemon juice*

Sort and rinse beans. Place beans and water in a Dutch oven. Soak overnight or boil 2 minutes; turn off heat and let stand for 1 hour before cooking. Do not drain.

Add ham and pepper; bring to a boil. Reduce heat, cover and simmer for about 2 hours or until beans are tender.

Add tomatoes with green chiles, salt, garlic, onion, and lemon juice. Cover and cook for 30 additional minutes over medium heat.

Serving size: 1 cup
Analysis per serving: 146 Calories, 10 g Protein, 26 g Carbohydrate,
1 g Fat, tr Sat Fat, % Calories from fat 6, 5 mg Cholesterol, 442 mg Sodium
Diabetic exchanges: 1 1/2 starches, 1/2 lean meat & 1 vegetable

NAVY BEAN SOUP

10 servings

3	cups dried navy beans
8	cups water
3	teaspoons chicken-flavored bouillon granules
1/2	teaspoon Italian seasoning
1/4	teaspoon dried minced garlic
1/4	teaspoon dried red pepper flakes
1	tablespoon olive oil
1	cup coarsely chopped green onions (tops included)

Sort and rinse beans. Place beans and water in a Dutch oven. Soak overnight or boil for 2 minutes; turn off heat and let stand for 1 hour before cooking. Do not drain.

Cover and simmer 2 hours or until beans are tender.

Add remaining ingredients; cover and cook for 20 additional minutes over medium heat.

Serving size: 1 cup
Analysis per serving: 176 Calories, 10 g Protein, 30 g Carbohydrate,
2 g Fat, tr Sat Fat, % Calories from fat 12, 0 mg Cholesterol, 272 mg Sodium
Diabetic exchanges: 2 starches & 1/2 lean meat

RED BEANS & GREENS SOUP

8 servings

2	cups red kidney beans
5	cups water
1	14 1/2-ounce can ready-to-serve chicken broth
2	ounces (1/2 cup) lean ham cubes
1/4	teaspoon dried minced garlic
1/4	teaspoon pepper
1/2	cup fresh or frozen chopped onion
1/4	teaspoon hot sauce
1	10-ounce box frozen chopped turnip greens
1/4	teaspoon salt

Sort and rinse kidney beans. Place kidney beans and water in a Dutch oven. Soak beans overnight or boil 2 minutes; turn off heat and let stand for 1 hour before cooking. Do not drain.

Add next 6 ingredients. Cover and bring to a boil; reduce heat and simmer for one hour. ☺

Add frozen greens and salt. Bring to a boil; reduce heat and simmer 15 minutes uncovered.

Serving size: 1 cup
Analysis per serving: 181 Calories, 14 g Protein, 30 g Carbohydrate,
1 g Fat, tr Sat Fat, % Calories from Fat 5, 4 mg Cholesterol, 385 mg Sodium
Diabetic exchanges: 1/2 lean meat, 2 starches & 1 vegetable

Split Pea Soup

7 servings

2	*cups dried green split peas*
1	*ounce (1/4 cup) chopped lean ham*
1	*14 1/2-ounce can ready-to-serve chicken broth*
1	*cup fresh or frozen chopped onion*
1/4	*teaspoon dried minced garlic*
1/4	*teaspoon pepper*
1/4	*teaspoon salt*
1/2	*teaspoon dried dillweed*

Place first six ingredients in a Dutch oven. Cover and simmer for 1 1/2 hours or until peas are tender. Stir in salt and dillweed. Serve hot.

Serving size: 1 cup
Analysis per serving: 217 Calories, 15 g Protein, 37 g Carbohydrate,
1 g Fat, tr Sat Fat, % Calories from fat 6, 2 mg Cholesterol, 389 mg Sodium
Diabetic exchanges: 2 1/2 starches & 1 lean meat

POTATO SOUP

See Figure 13 (page 61) for use of a scrubber attached to the sink.
6 servings

6	medium-sized new potatoes, unpeeled and scrubbed
3	cups water
2	tablespoons dried minced onion
1	cup frozen sliced carrots
1	cup celery, coarsely chopped
2	teaspoons chicken-flavored bouillon granules
1/4	teaspoon thyme
1	bay leaf
1/2	cup evaporated skim milk
1	cup skim milk

Place first 8 ingredients in a Dutch oven. Cover and cook over medium heat until potatoes are tender.

Remove potatoes from soup with a fork or slotted spoon. Place on a cutting board and allow to cool slightly before handling. Cut potatoes into quarters and return to soup mixture. ☺

Stir in evaporated milk and skim milk. Cook over low heat, stirring frequently, until mixture is thoroughly heated (do not boil). Remove bay leaf before serving.

Serving size: 1 cup
Analysis per serving: 133 Calories, 6 g Protein, 27 g Carbohydrate,
1 g Fat, tr Sat Fat, % Calories from Fat 7, 2 mg Cholesterol, 392 mg Sodium
Diabetic exchanges: 1 1/2 starches & 1/2 vegetable

Salads

Contents

FIESTA RICE SALAD

8 servings

1 1/4	cups water
1/2	cup uncooked rice
1	15-ounce can black beans, rinsed and drained
1	11-ounce can no-salt-added corn kernels, drained
2	teaspoons dried minced onion
2	tablespoons chopped green chiles
1/4	cup fresh or frozen chopped green pepper
Dash garlic powder	
1	2-ounce jar chopped pimento, drained

Dressing

1/4	cup nonfat plain yogurt
1	tablespoon lemon juice
3/4	teaspoon ground cumin
Dash ground pepper	

Combine water and rice in a medium saucepan. Cover and bring to a boil; reduce heat, and simmer 25 minutes or until liquid is absorbed.

Combine rice and remaining ingredients in a 2-quart bowl, tossing gently to combine.

To make dressing: stir together yogurt, lemon juice, cumin, and pepper. Pour over rice mixture and toss again to mix.

Cover and refrigerate until ready to serve.

Serving size: 1/2 cup
Analysis per serving: 136 Calories, 5 g Protein, 28 g Carbohydrate,
1 g Fat, tr Sat Fat, % Calories from Fat 7, tr Cholesterol, 192 mg Sodium
Diabetic exchanges: 2 starches

PASTA SALAD PRIMAVERA

You can buy broccoli florets and other prepared vegetables
on the salad bar at some supermarkets.
6 servings

1	cup corkscrew-shaped pasta
1 1/2	cups raw broccoli florets
1/4	cup sliced green onions
1	cup quartered cherry tomatoes
1/4	cup reduced-fat Italian dressing
1/4	teaspoon salt

Cook pasta according to package directions, omitting salt or fat. Drain well
and cool. Place in a large bowl and add remaining ingredients. Toss well to
coat. Cover and chill.

Serving size: 3/4 cup
Analysis per serving: 124 Calories, 4 g Protein, 24 g Carbohydrate,
2 g Fat, 0 g Sat Fat, % Calories from Fat 14, 0 mg Cholesterol, 253 mg Sodium
Diabetic exchanges: 1 starch & 2 vegetables

COTTAGE CHEESE SALAD

5 servings

1/2	*cup chopped green pepper*
1/2	*cup chopped cucumber, unpeeled*
1	*tablespoon chopped green onion (including tops)*
1/2	*cup cherry tomatoes, cut into halves*
1	*16-ounce carton low-fat cottage cheese*
5	*lettuce leaves*

Stir prepared vegetables into cottage cheese. Serve on lettuce leaves

Variation: Add sliced radishes, chopped celery or diced yellow squash.

Serving size: 1/2 cup
Analysis per serving: 73 Calories, 11 g Protein, 4 g Carbohydrate,
1 g Fat, 1 g Sat Fat, % Calories from Fat 12, 4 mg Cholesterol, 371 mg Sodium
Diabetic exchanges: 1 lean meat & 1 vegetable

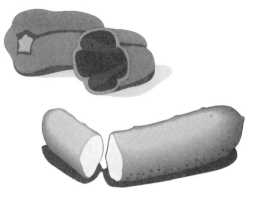

COTTAGE CHEESE
& FRUIT SALAD PLATE

Kiwis can be cut in half and eaten from the skin with a spoon.
There is no need to peel the fruit.

2 salads

2	*large lettuce leaves*
2	*bananas, sliced lengthwise*
1/2	*cup fresh strawberries, halved*
4	*1/2-inch slices fresh pineapple, cored and peeled*
1	*cup low-fat cottage cheese*
2	*kiwis, unpeeled and halved*
1	*11-ounce can mandarin oranges, drained*
2	*tablespoons commercial poppyseed dressing*

Equally divide fruit and cottage cheese. Arrange on lettuce leaves.

Drizzle each salad with 1 tablespoon poppyseed dressing.

Serving size: 1/2 cup cottage cheese, 1/2 of fruit mixture and 1 tablespoon dressing
Analysis per serving: 384 Calories, 14 g Protein, 74 g Carbohydrate,
7 g Fat, 1 g Sat Fat, % Calories from Fat 16, 4 mg Cholesterol, 349 mg Sodium
Diabetic exchanges: 5 fruits, 2 lean meats & 1/2 fat

BLUEBERRY, PEACH & GRAPE SALAD

9 servings

1	16-ounce can sliced peaches, packed in juice
Water	with peach liquid to equal 1 cup
1	3-ounce package lemon- or peach-flavored gelatin
1	cup cold water
1/2	cup seedless grapes
1	cup fresh or frozen blueberries

Dressing

1/4	cup fat-free sour cream
1/4	cup reduced-calorie mayonnaise

Drain peaches and reserve liquid in a measuring cup.

Add water to peach liquid until it measures 1 cup and place in a small saucepan. Cover and heat to boiling.

Remove from heat and add gelatin, stirring until dissolved. Add 1 cup cold water and pour into a 9-inch square dish. Chill until slightly thickened.

Add peaches, grapes, and blueberries. Stir gently to combine. Cover and chill until set.

Combine dressing ingredients in a small bowl, and spread dressing evenly over gelatin. Cut into 9 squares.

Serving size: 1 square
Analysis per serving: 100 Calories, 2 g Protein, 19 g Carbohydrate,
2 g Fat, tr Sat Fat, 1 mg Cholesterol, 86 mg Sodium
Diabetic exchanges: 1/2 starch & 1 fruit

MANDARIN ORANGE
GELATIN SALAD

Keep pliers in the kitchen for tasks you find difficult,
such as removing the opener strip on a can of orange juice.
9 servings

1	*8-ounce can unsweetened crushed pineapple*
1	*11-ounce can mandarin oranges*
Water	*with juice from fruit to equal 1 1/4 cups*
1	*3-ounce package orange-flavored gelatin*
1	*6-ounce can frozen orange juice concentrate, thawed*

Drain fruits and set aside, reserving liquids in a measuring cup. Add water to combined liquids until it measures 1 1/4 cup and place in a small saucepan. Cover and heat to boiling.

Remove from heat and add gelatin, stirring until dissolved. Add orange juice concentrate and stir. Cool until slightly thickened.

Add fruits and gently stir to combine. Pour into a 9-inch square dish; cover and chill until set. Cut into 9 portions.

Serving size: 1 square
Analysis per serving: 95 Calories, 2 g Protein, 23 g Carbohydrate,
tr Fat, tr Sat Fat, 0 mg Cholesterol, 31 mg Sodium
Diabetic exchanges: 1 fruit & 1/2 starch

CRANBERRY SALAD

9 servings

3/4	*cup water*
1	*3-ounce package cherry-flavored gelatin*
1	*12-ounce jar cranberry-orange fruit mixture*
1/4	*cup chopped celery*
1	*8-ounce can unsweetened crushed pineapple, undrained*
2	*tablespoons chopped pecans*

Place water in a small saucepan; cover and heat to boiling. Remove from heat; add gelatin, stirring until dissolved. Cool until slightly thickened.

Add remaining ingredients and pour into a 9-inch square dish. Cover and chill until set. Cut into 9 squares.

Serving size: 1 square
Analysis per serving: 132 Calories, 1 g Protein, 30 g Carbohydrate,
1 g Fat, tr Sat Fat, 0 mg Cholesterol, 45 mg Sodium
Diabetic exchanges: 1 fruit & 1 starch

FRESH FRUIT SALAD

Canned unsweetened pineapple chunks may be substituted
if fresh, pared pineapple is not available.
6 servings

1 1/2   *cups fresh strawberries, halved*
1 1/2   *cups seedless grapes*
1   *cup fresh pineapple chunks*
1   *cup chopped pears*
2   *medium-sized bananas*

Dressing *(makes 3/4 cup)*
3/4   *cup vanilla low-fat yogurt*
2   *teaspoons lemon juice*
Dash nutmeg

Place prepared fruit except banana in a large bowl. Just before serving, slice bananas and add to fruit mixture. Toss fruit lightly to mix. Divide into 6 servings.

Combine dressing ingredients in a small bowl, and drizzle 2 tablespoons of dressing over each salad before serving.

Hint: Dip sliced bananas in pineapple or orange juice to prevent browning.

Serving size: 1 cup fruit with 2 tablespoons dressing
Analysis per serving: 122 Calories, 3 g Protein, 28 g Carbohydrate,
1 g Fat, tr Sat Fat, 2 mg Cholesterol, 22 mg Sodium
Diabetic exchanges: 2 fruits

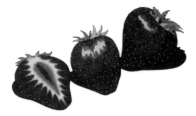

FROZEN FRUIT SALAD

8 servings

1	16-ounce can fruit cocktail in light syrup, drained
1/2	cup vanilla low-fat yogurt
1	cup miniature marshmallows
2	tablespoons fat-free mayonnaise
2	tablespoons orange juice

Lettuce leaves

Mix drained fruit with yogurt, marshmallows, mayonnaise, and orange juice.

Spoon into foil cupcake liners which have been placed in muffin pans. Cover with plastic wrap and freeze overnight.

To serve, peel off foil cupcake liners and place on lettuce leaves. (You may need to let frozen salads set out about 5 minutes before removing foil). Salads should sit out at room temperature 30 to 40 minutes to soften slightly before serving.

Serving size: 1/3 cup
Analysis per serving: 83 Calories, 1 g Protein, 20 g Carbohydrate,
tr Fat, tr Sat Fat, 2 mg Cholesterol, 44 mg Sodium
Diabetic exchanges: 1 1/2 fruits

CELERY CABBAGE SALAD

Fresh bean sprouts may be added,
and it can be covered and stored overnight in the refrigerator.
8 servings

1	*bunch Chinese celery cabbage (bok choy)*
1	*tablespoon sugar*
2	*tablespoons cider vinegar*
1	*tablespoon water*
2	*teaspoons reduced-sodium soy sauce*

Wash Chinese cabbage stalks and slice across ribs. Place in a 1 1/2-quart bowl and set aside.

Combine sugar, vinegar, water and soy sauce in a small bowl, stirring until sugar is dissolved. Pour vinegar mixture over cabbage and toss.

Cover and refrigerate until ready to serve.

Serving size: 1/2 cup
Analysis per serving: 24 Calories, 1 g Protein, 5 g Carbohydrate,
tr Fat, tr Sat Fat, 0 mg Cholesterol, 114 mg Sodium
Diabetic exchange: 1 vegetable

Citrus Spinach Salad

Leaf lettuce may be substituted for spinach.

4 servings

1	small, red onion
6	cups fresh spinach
1	16-ounce can grapefruit sections, drained (reserve 1/2 cup juice)
1/4	cup plain croutons

Citrus Vinaigrette *(makes 3/4 cup)*

1	tablespoon corn oil
1	tablespoon Dijon mustard
1/2	cup grapefruit juice (reserved from canned grapefruit sections)
1/4	teaspoon paprika
1/4	teaspoon pepper
1/4	teaspoon salt
1	tablespoon sugar

Slice onion and separate into rings. Tear spinach into bite-size pieces. Combine onion, spinach and grapefruit sections in a large serving bowl. Cover and refrigerate until ready to serve. Top with croutons. Serve vinaigrette separately.

Combine all ingredients in a small bowl, stirring well to dissolve sugar. Cover and refrigerate until dressing is thoroughly chilled.

Serving size: 2 cups salad and 3 tablespoons vinaigrette
Analysis per serving: 110 Calories, 4 g Protein, 18 g Carbohydrate,
4 g Fat, tr Sat Fat, 0 mg Cholesterol, 260 mg Sodium
Diabetic exchanges: 1 fruit, 1/2 vegetable & 1 fat

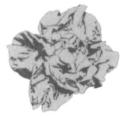

COLESLAW

5 servings

2 1/2	*cups shredded cabbage*
1/4	*cup coarsely chopped cucumber, unpeeled*
2	*tablespoons vinegar*
1	*tablespoon sugar*
1	*tablespoon water*
1/4	*teaspoon salt*

Place cabbage and cucumber in a large bowl. Set aside.

Combine vinegar, sugar, water and salt in a small bowl. Stir to dissolve sugar. Pour over vegetables, and toss gently to combine.

Cover and chill 30 minutes before serving.

Serving size: 1/2 cup
Analysis per serving: 19 Calories, tr Protein, 5 g Carbohydrate,
tr Fat, tr Sat Fat, 0 mg Cholesterol, 104 mg Sodium
Diabetic exchange: 1 vegetable

Green Pea Salad

4 servings

1	10-ounce package frozen small green peas*
1/3	cup chopped celery
2	tablespoons sweet pickle relish
1/3	cup shredded reduced-fat Cheddar cheese
2	tablespoons reduced-calorie mayonnaise

Cook peas according to package directions omitting salt and margarine. Remove from heat, drain and cool.

Combine all ingredients in a bowl. Cover and chill before serving.

* Drained, canned peas may be used.

Serving size: 1/2 cup
Analysis per serving: 116 Calories, 6 g Protein, 13 g Carbohydrate,
5 g Fat, 2 g Sat Fat, 6 mg Cholesterol, 252 mg Sodium
Diabetic exchanges: 1 starch & 1/2 medium-fat meat

MARINATED CARROT SALAD

This is best made ahead of time. It will keep for a week in the refrigerator.
6 servings

1	*10 3/4-ounce can (1/3 less salt, 99% fat-free) tomato soup*
1/3	*cup sugar*
1/4	*cup vinegar*
1	*teaspoon prepared mustard*
1	*teaspoon low-sodium Worcestershire sauce*
1	*cup frozen chopped onion*
1	*cup frozen chopped green pepper*
1	*16-ounce can sliced carrots, drained*

Combine first 5 ingredients in a medium bowl. Blend with a spoon or hand-held mixer until sugar dissolves.

Add vegetables and toss gently to coat. Cover and chill. Serve with a slotted spoon.

Serving size: 1/2 cup
Analysis per serving: 58 Calories, 1 g Protein, 13 g Carbohydrate,
1 g Fat, tr Sat Fat, 0 g Cholesterol, 224 mg Sodium
Diabetic exchanges: 1/2 starch & 1 vegetable

YOGURT POTATO SALAD

8 servings

2	*pounds new potatoes, unpeeled and scrubbed*
3	*green onions, chopped (including tops)*
1	*tablespoon Dijon mustard*
3/4	*cup plain nonfat yogurt*
1/2	*teaspoon salt*

Dash pepper

1/2	*teaspoon celery seed*

Place potatoes in Dutch oven, add water to cover. Bring to a boil, reduce heat and simmer 30 minutes, or until potatoes are tender.

Remove potatoes from water with a fork or slotted spoon. Place on a cutting board and allow to cool slightly before handling. Cut potatoes into quarters. Set aside.

Combine onions, mustard, yogurt, salt, pepper and celery seed in a large bowl, mixing well. Add potatoes and stir gently to coat. May be served warm or chilled.

Serving size: 1/2 cup
Analysis per serving: 114 Calories, 4 g Protein, 25 g Carbohydrate,
tr Fat, tr Saturated Fat, tr Cholesterol, 167 mg Sodium
Diabetic exchanges: 1 1/2 starches

Main Dishes

Contents

BROCCOLI RICE CASSEROLE

This makes a great vegetarian entree.
4 servings

2 1/2	cups water
1	cup uncooked brown rice
1	teaspoon margarine
2	cups pre-sliced fresh mushrooms
1	teaspoon chicken-flavored bouillon granules
1/4	teaspoon salt
2	tablespoons dehydrated onion flakes
1/4	teaspoon dried minced garlic
1/8	teaspoon pepper
1/2	teaspoon dried Italian seasoning
1	10-ounce package frozen broccoli florets
1/2	cup shredded reduced-fat Monterey Jack cheese
2	tablespoons chopped pecans

Combine water, rice, margarine, mushrooms, chicken granules, salt, onion flakes, garlic, pepper, and Italian seasoning in a medium saucepan. Cover and bring to a boil; reduce heat and simmer 35 minutes.☺

Add broccoli florets. Cover and continue cooking for 20 minutes or until rice has absorbed water and broccoli is crisp-tender.

Top with grated cheese and chopped pecans.

Serving size: 1 1/2 cups
Analysis per serving: 288 Calories, 12 g Protein, 46 g Carbohydrate,
8 g Fat, 2 g Sat Fat, % Calories from Fat 25, 9 mg Cholesterol, 461 mg Sodium
Diabetic exchanges: 1/2 lean meat, 2 1/2 starches, 1 vegetable & 1 fat

BROCCOLI-TOPPED POTATOES

Potatoes and broccoli may be cooked in a microwave oven.
4 servings

4	*large baking potatoes, unpeeled and scrubbed*
1	*10-ounce package frozen broccoli florets*
4	*teaspoons margarine*
1/4	*cup fat-free sour cream*
1/2	*cup shredded reduced-fat sharp Cheddar cheese*
2	*green onions, chopped (including tops)*

Prick each potato 3 times with tip of a knife. Bake at 400° for 1 hour or until potatoes are tender. ☺

During last 15 minutes of cooking time, cook broccoli according to package directions without added salt.

Cut slit in top of each potato. Top each potato evenly with margarine, broccoli, fat-free sour cream, cheese and green onion.

Serving size: 1 potato
Analysis per serving: 413 Calories, 14 g Protein, 76 g Carbohydrate,
7 g Fat, 2 g Sat Fat, % Calories from Fat 15, 9 mg Cholesterol, 189 mg Sodium
Diabetic exchanges: 4 1/2 starches, 1 vegetable & 1 fat

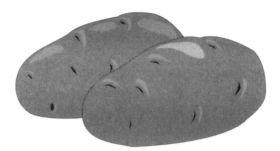

Potato Cheese Frittata

4 servings

Vegetable cooking spray
1   cup frozen hash brown potatoes
1/2   cup chopped fresh or frozen onion
1/2   cup chopped fresh or frozen green pepper
1   cup egg substitute
1/2   teaspoon low-sodium Worcestershire sauce
1/4   teaspoon hot sauce
1/4   teaspoon salt
1/4   cup shredded reduced-fat Cheddar cheese

Spray a 10-inch nonstick skillet with cooking spray. Heat skillet over medium heat and add potatoes. Spread potatoes evenly in skillet. Cover and cook 5 minutes. Remove cover and stir.

Add onion and green pepper to potatoes. Cover and cook 5 minutes. ☺

Mix egg substitute with Worcestershire, hot sauce and salt. Pour over potato mixture, and continue cooking over medium heat until egg is nearly set.

Top with cheese. Cover and cook until cheese is melted and egg is set on top. Cut into 4 wedges.

Serving size: 1 wedge
Analysis per serving: 114 Calories, 10 g Protein, 15 g Carbohydrate,
2 g Fat, 1 g Sat Fat, % Calories from Fat 16, 5 mg Cholesterol, 326 mg Sodium
Diabetic exchanges: 1 starch, 1/4 vegetable & 1 lean meat

RED BEANS & RICE

7 servings

6	*cups water*
2 1/2	*cups dried red kidney beans*
4	*ounces (1 cup) lean ham, chopped*
1	*cup frozen chopped onion*
1	*bay leaf*
1/2	*teaspoon salt*
1/4	*teaspoon pepper*
1	*teaspoon hot sauce*
3 1/2	*cups cooked rice (cooked without salt or fat)*

Sort and rinse beans. Place water and beans in a Dutch oven. Soak overnight or boil two minutes; turn off heat and let stand 1 hour before cooking. Do not drain.

Add ham, onion and bay leaf. Cover and bring to a boil; reduce heat and simmer for 1 hour or until beans are tender.

Add remaining ingredients (except rice) and stir. Remove bay leaf.

To serve, place 1/2 cup hot rice in a bowl and top with 1 cup bean mixture.

Serving size: 1/2 cup rice plus 1 cup beans
Analysis per serving: 341 Calories, 20 g Protein, 62 g Carbohydrate,
1 g Fat, tr Sat Fat, % Calories from Fat 4, 7 mg Cholesterol, 398 mg Sodium
Diabetic exchanges: 4 starches & 1 lean meat

MAIN DISH MEXICAN CASSEROLE

4 servings

2	*cups dried kidney beans*
3 1/4	*cups water, divided*
1/2	*cup uncooked brown rice*
1	*28-ounce can crushed tomatoes*
1	*tablespoon dried onion*
1	*teaspoon paprika*
1/2	*cup shredded reduced-fat sharp Cheddar cheese*

Wash and sort beans; place in a large Dutch oven. Cover with water 2 inches above beans and soak overnight; drain. Add 2 cups water to Dutch oven and cook for 1 hour or until tender. Drain beans well. ☺

Cook rice in 1 1/4 cups water for 45 minutes.

Add cooked rice, tomatoes, onion, and paprika to beans. Bring bean mixture to a boil; remove from heat and top with cheese. Serve from Dutch oven.

Serving size: 1 cup
Analysis per serving: 262 Calories, 15 g Protein, 41 g Carbohydrate,
5 g Fat, 2 g Sat Fat, % Calories from Fat 17, 9 mg Cholesterol, 503 mg Sodium
Diabetic exchanges: 2 1/2 starches, 1 vegetable & 1/2 medium-fat meat

Mushroom Lasagna

This recipe was divided into two pans for ease in lifting.
A 9" x 13" pan is also appropriate.
8 servings

Tomato Sauce

1/4	cup frozen chopped onion
1	pound fresh sliced mushrooms
1	12-ounce can crushed tomatoes
1	6-ounce can tomato paste
1	cup low-sodium beef-flavored bouillon cubes

Ricotta Sauce

1	cup fat-free Ricotta cheese
1	egg
1/8	teaspoon pepper
2	tablespoons fresh grated Parmesan cheese

	Vegetable cooking spray
12	uncooked whole wheat lasagna noodles
2	cups grated light Mozzarella cheese
1/4	cup fresh grated Parmesan cheese

Place all tomato sauce ingredients in a Dutch oven over medium heat. Cover and simmer for 30 minutes. In a medium-sized bowl, beat all Ricotta sauce ingredients together with a wire wisk. ☺

Spray two 8-inch square pans with cooking spray. Layer lasagna ingredients in each pan. Start with 3 lasagna noodles. Top noodles with 1 cup tomato sauce, then half the Ricotta mixture. Sprinkle 1/2 cup mozzarella over Ricotta.

Add 3 more lasagna noodles. Top with 1 cup sauce. Sprinkle 1/2 cup mozzarella and 2 tablespoons Parmesan over tomato sauce layer.

Cover pans with foil and place in refrigerator overnight. Bake at 350° for 1 hour. Uncover and bake for 10 additional minutes or until lightly browned.

Cut each pan into 4 squares.

Variation: Add a 10-ounce package of frozen, chopped, drained spinach to the middle layer.

Serving size: 1/4 pan
Analysis per serving: 226 Calories, 19 g Protein, 27 g Carbohydrate,
7 g Fat, 1 g Sat Fat, % of Calories from Fat 28, 49 mg Cholesterol, 512 mg Sodium
Diabetic exchanges: 2 starches & 2 lean meats

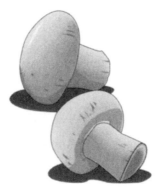

VEGETARIAN PIZZA

Prepared pizza crust is available unbaked in the refrigerated section
of larger supermarkets. If your supermarket has a salad bar,
you may wish to purchase onion, green pepper, and mushrooms there.
8 servings

1	*12-inch refrigerated prepared pizza crust*
1	*cup prepared pizza sauce*
1/2	*cup chopped onion*
1	*medium green pepper, chopped*
2	*cups fresh sliced mushrooms*
1	*cup shredded part-skim mozzarella cheese*

Preheat oven 450°. Spread pizza sauce on crust placed on a cookie sheet.
Sprinkle remaining ingredients over sauce in the order listed. Bake 10 to 12
minutes or until crust is golden and cheese is melted.

Serving size: 1 slice
Analysis per serving: 269 Calories, 10 g Protein, 42 Carbohydrate,
7 g Fat, 2 g Sat Fat, % Calories from Fat 22, 8 mg Cholesterol, 487 mg Sodium
Diabetic exchanges: 2 1/2 starches, 1 vegetable, 1/2 medium-fat meat & 1 fat

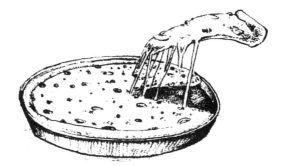

BAKED CATFISH

4 servings

4   4-ounce catfish fillets
Vegetable cooking spray
3   *tablespoons lemon juice*
1/4   *cup yellow cornmeal*
1/2   *teaspoon lemon pepper*

Preheat oven to 400°. Place fish fillets in a 9-inch square baking pan which has been coated with cooking spray. Drizzle lemon juice over fish.

Sprinkle 1 tablespoon cornmeal over each fish fillet, turning to coat each side. Sprinkle lemon pepper evenly over fish.

Bake 15 to 20 minutes or until fish flakes easily when tested with a fork.

Serving size: 1 fillet
Analysis per serving: 171 Calories, 21 g Protein, 9 g Carbohydrate,
5 g Fat, 1 g Sat Fat, % Calories from Fat 27, 65 mg Cholesterol, 219 mg Sodium
Diabetic exchanges: 1/2 starch & 2 1/2 lean meats

BAKED ORANGE ROUGHY

4 servings

Olive oil cooking spray
4   4-ounce orange roughy fillets
2   tablespoons lemon juice
1/4   teaspoon salt
3   tablespoons Italian-seasoned breadcrumbs
Lemon wedges

Coat an 8-inch square baking pan with olive oil cooking spray. Place fish fillets in the pan and drizzle with lemon juice.

Sprinkle salt and breadcrumbs evenly over fillets. Coat fish fillets lightly with olive oil cooking spray.

Bake at 350° for 20 minutes or until fish flakes easily with a fork. Broil 1 minute to lightly brown crumbs, if desired. Garnish with lemon wedges.

Serving size: 1 fillet
Analysis per serving: 129 Calories, 22 g Protein, 4 g Carbohydrate,
2 g Fat, tr Sat Fat, % Calories from Fat 12, 63 mg Cholesterol, 269 mg Sodium
Diabetic exchanges: 1/4 starch & 3 lean meats

BAKED SALMON
WITH CUCUMBER SAUCE

4 servings

Vegetable cooking spray
4	*4-ounce salmon steaks*
1	*teaspoon margarine, melted*
1/4	*teaspoon salt*
1/4	*teaspoon pepper*

Cucumber Sauce
1/2	*cup peeled and grated cucumber*
2	*tablespoons reduced-calorie mayonnaise*
2	*tablespoons fat-free sour cream*

Preheat oven to 400°. Coat a baking dish or pan with cooking spray. Rinse salmon steaks and pat dry with paper towels.

Place salmon in coated baking pan. Evenly spread the melted margarine over the fish. Sprinkle with salt and pepper.

Bake for 20 minutes or until fish flakes when tested with a fork. ☺

Mix cucumber sauce ingredients in a small bowl. Top each steak with 3 tablespoons cucumber sauce before serving.

Serving size: 1 salmon steak with 3 tablespoons cucumber sauce
Analysis per serving: 217 Calories, 24 g Protein, 3 g Carbohydrate,
11 g Fat, 4 g Sat Fat, % Calories from Fat 47, 77 mg Cholesterol, 275 mg Sodium
Diabetic exchanges: 3 lean meats & 1 fat

ORANGE ROUGHY
WITH LEMON-BASIL SAUCE

4 servings

4   *4-ounce orange roughy fillets*
Paprika

Lemon-Basil Sauce
1   teaspoon margarine
2   teaspoons all-purpose flour
1/2   cup skim milk
2   teaspoons lemon juice
1/8   teaspoon dried crushed basil
1/4   teaspoon salt

Place fillets in a baking dish; sprinkle with paprika. Bake at 400° for 15 to 20 minutes or until fish flakes easily when tested with a fork.☺

To make sauce, melt margarine in a small saucepan on medium heat. Blend in flour with a wire whisk. Add milk and stir until mixture thickens. Remove from heat and stir in lemon juice, basil, and salt.

Top each baked fillet with 2 tablespoons of sauce.

Serving size: 1 fish fillet and 2 tablespoons sauce
Analysis per serving: 132 Calories, 24 g Protein, 3 g Carbohydrate,
2 g Fat, 1 g Sat Fat, % Calories from Fat 17, 63 mg Cholesterol, 257 mg Sodium
Diabetic exchanges: 1/4 starch & 3 lean meats

SHRIMP REMOULADE WITH PASTA

3 servings

1 1/2	cups bowtie-shaped pasta
1/4	cup reduced-fat mayonnaise
2	tablespoons chopped fresh parsley
1/4	cup sliced green onions
1	tablespoon white wine vinegar
1/2	teaspoon Worcestershire sauce
1/4	teaspoon paprika
1/4	teaspoon salt
1/2	pound cooked, shelled, deveined shrimp

Cook pasta according to package directions, omitting salt or fat. Drain well and cool. Set aside.

Combine mayonnaise, parsley, green onions, vinegar, Worcestershire sauce, paprika, and salt in a large bowl.

Add pasta and shrimp, tossing to coat. Cover and chill.

Serving size: 1 cup
Analysis per serving: 260 Calories, 20 g Protein, 26 g Carbohydrate,
8 g Fat, tr Sat Fat, % Calories from Fat 29, 153 mg Cholesterol, 507 mg Sodium
Diabetic exchanges: 2 starches, 2 lean meats & 1 fat

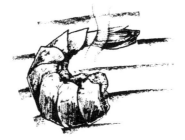

SHRIMP WITH PASTA

6 servings

3	cups cooked multicolored corkscrew-shaped pasta (1 1/2 cups uncooked)
1	tablespoon margarine
1	cup sliced green onions
1	cup sliced fresh mushrooms
1/4	teaspoon dry minced garlic
1	teaspoon lemon juice
1	teaspoon chicken broth granules
1	tablespoon cornstarch
1	cup water
1	pound cooked, shelled, deveined shrimp
1	cup fat-free sour cream
	Vegetable cooking spray
1/2	cup shredded reduced-fat Cheddar cheese

Cook pasta in unsalted water according to package directions or until tender but not soft. Drain.

Melt margarine in nonstick skillet. Add sliced green onions and mushrooms. Saute over medium heat for 2 to 3 minutes, stirring as needed. Add garlic, lemon juice, and chicken granules.

Stir cornstarch into cold water with a fork or wire whisk and add to onion/mushroom mixture. Cook over medium heat until thickened, stirring as needed to prevent sticking. Add shrimp and cook 2 to 3 minutes or until shrimp is hot. Remove from heat and stir in fat-free sour cream. Add cooked pasta and stir gently.

Spoon or pour into a 2-quart casserole dish which has been lightly coated with cooking spray. Top with shredded cheese. Heat in a 350° oven until cheese is melted.

Serving size: 1 cup
Analysis per serving: 260 Calories, 20 g Protein, 26 g Carbohydrate,
8 g Fat, 1 g Sat Fat, % Calories from Fat 28, 153 mg Cholesterol, 507 mg Sodium
Diabetic exchanges: 1 1/2 starches, 1/2 vegetable, 2 lean meats & 1/2 fat

TUNA CROQUETTES
WITH RATATOUILLE

4 servings

1   12-ounce can tuna, packed in water
1   egg white
1   tablespoon chopped onion
1/2 cup cracker crumbs
Vegetable cooking spray

Ratatouille
1   cup chopped tomato
1   cup chopped, unpeeled eggplant
1/4 cup chopped green pepper
1/8 teaspoon salt
1   tablespoon olive oil

Drain tuna and combine with the next 3 ingredients. Form into flat cakes
and place in a skillet coated lightly with cooking spray.

Cook over medium heat until brown on both sides, turning once (approximately 4 minutes on each side). ☺

Combine all ratatouille ingredients in a nonstick skillet. Cover and bring
mixture to a gentle boil over medium heat, stirring once or twice. Reduce
heat and cook covered for 10 minutes or until vegetables are tender.

Top each croquette with 1/2 cup of vegetable mixture.

Servings size: 1 tuna croquette with 1/2 cup vegetable topping
Analysis per serving: 203 Calories, 27 g Protein, 10 g Carbohydrate,
5 g Fat, 1 g Saturated Fat, % Calories from Fat 24, 16 mg Cholesterol, 498 mg Sodium
Diabetic exchanges: 3 lean meats & 2 vegetables

CHICKEN & RICE SALAD

8 ounces (1/2 pound) skinless chicken breasts
yields approximately 1 1/4 cups cooked chicken.
6 servings

1	*6.9-ounce package chicken-flavored Rice-A-Roni® cooked by package directions without added fat*
1 1/4	*cups chopped cooked chicken breast (skinned before cooking and cooked without salt)*
1	*2 1/4-ounce can sliced ripe olives*
1	*6 1/2-ounce jar artichoke hearts, marinated in oil mixture and finely chopped*
1	*8-ounce can sliced water chestnuts, drained*
1/2	*cup chopped red pepper*

Mix all prepared ingredients, including artichoke marinade, in a medium bowl, stirring gently until well blended. Serve hot or cover and refrigerate before serving cold.

Serving size: 1 cup
Analysis per serving: 146 Calories, 12 g Protein, 18 g Carbohydrate,
3 g Fat, 1 g Sat Fat, % Calories from Fat 21, 23 mg Cholesterol, 427 mg Sodium
Diabetic exchanges: 1 starch, 1/2 vegetable & 1 lean meat

CHICKEN &
SUMMER VEGETABLES

2 servings

1	cup water
1	teaspoon chicken-flavored bouillon granules
2	tablespoons dried onion

Dash garlic salt

1/2	cup rice, uncooked
1	cup frozen sliced carrots
8	ounces boneless, skinless chicken breasts

1	small yellow squash, cut into halves
1	medium zucchini, cut into halves
1	6-inch piece celery, cut into halves

Combine first 4 ingredients in a saucepan. Cover and bring to a boil.

Stir in rice. Place carrots, then chicken breasts on rice. Reduce heat and simmer, covered, for 10 minutes. ☺

Place yellow squash, zucchini, and celery on chicken and continue cooking, covered, an additional 15 minutes or until chicken and vegetables are tender. Do not stir after adding chicken and vegetables.

Serve from pan.

Serving size: 1 portion
Analysis per serving: 334 Calories, 32 g Protein, 43 g Carbohydrate,
4 g Fat, 1 g Sat Fat, % Calories from Fat 9, 71 mg Cholesterol, 536 mg Sodium
Diabetic exchanges: 2 starches, 2 vegetables & 3 lean meats

CHICKEN DIVAN

6 servings

1	*pound bag frozen chopped broccoli*
1	*pound (6 pieces) boneless, skinless chicken breasts*
1	*can 99% fat-free mushroom soup*
1/4	*cup light sour cream*
1/2	*cup shredded reduced-fat sharp Cheddar cheese*
1/4	*cup sliced almonds*

Evenly place frozen broccoli in a 9-x 13-x 2-inch baking dish. Lay chicken breasts on broccoli.

Combine mushroom soup and sour cream in a small bowl, and spread over the chicken and broccoli. Sprinkle cheese and almonds over the top.

Bake uncovered at 350° for 1 hour.

Serving size: 1 chicken breast with 1/6 of broccoli and sauce
Analysis per serving: 216 Calories, 23 g Protein, 10 g Carbohydrate,
10 g Fat, 4 g Sat Fat, % Calories from Fat 30, 46 mg Cholesterol, 325 mg Sodium
Diabetic exchanges: 1/2 starch, 1 vegetable & 3 lean meats

CRISPY BAKED CHICKEN

4 servings

1	*pound boneless, skinless chicken breasts*
2	*tablespoons skim milk*
1	*teaspoon lemon pepper*
1/2	*teaspoon paprika*
1/4	*teaspoon thyme*
1/2	*cup breadcrumbs*

Vegetable cooking spray

Brush chicken breasts with milk, and sprinkle each piece evenly with lemon pepper, paprika and thyme. Dredge chicken pieces in breadcrumbs.

Place a cooking rack in a baking pan and coat with cooking spray. Place chicken on the rack and lightly coat chicken with cooking spray.

Bake at 400º for 15 to 20 minutes until tender and juices are clear. Broil for 1 minute to lightly brown chicken if desired.

Serving size: 1 chicken breast
Analysis per serving: 169 Calories, 17 g Protein, 5 g Carbohydrate,
3 g Fat, 1 g Sat Fat, % Calories from Fat 18, 72 mg Cholesterol, 131 mg Sodium
Diabetic exchanges: 1/4 starch & 2 1/2 lean meats

FAJITAS

For a "spicier" marinade, add 1/4 teaspoon cumin.
10 servings

1	*tablespoon Worcestershire sauce*
1	*teaspoon lemon juice*
1/4	*teaspoon salt*
1	*pound boneless, skinless chicken breasts cut into 1/2-inch strips*

	Vegetable cooking spray
1	*medium onion, sliced*
1	*medium green pepper, sliced*
10	*flour tortillas*
10	*tablespoons fat-free sour cream*
10	*tablespoons commercial salsa*

Combine Worcestershire sauce, lemon juice, and salt in a small bowl. Add chicken and stir to coat. Cover and place in the refrigerator for 30 minutes.☺

Coat a large nonstick skillet with cooking spray and place over medium heat. Add chicken to hot skillet and stir-fry about 7 minutes, or until chicken is no longer pink and is tender. Remove chicken from skillet, and set aside.

Add onion and green pepper to remaining juices in the skillet; stir-fry 3 minutes. Return chicken to skillet. Stir-fry 1 minute or until thoroughly heated. Place 1/2 cup chicken and vegetable mixture on a tortilla and top with 1 tablespoon fat-free sour cream and 1 tablespoon salsa. Roll tortilla around filling and serve immediately.

Serving size: 1 tortilla, 1/2 cup chicken and vegetable mixture
and 1 tablespoon each of fat-free sour cream and salsa.
Analysis per serving: 207 Calories, 14 g Protein, 26 g Carbohydrate,
6 g Fat, 3 g Sat Fat, % Calories from Fat 27, 28 mg Cholesterol, 361 mg Sodium
Diabetic exchanges: 1 1/2 starches, 1/2 vegetable, 1 lean meat & 1/2 fat

HERBED CHICKEN

6 servings

1	*pound boneless, skinless chicken breasts*
2	*teaspoons olive oil*
Olive oil vegetable cooking spray	
1	*tablespoon lemon juice*
1/2	*teaspoon rosemary*
1/4	*teaspoon salt*
1/4	*teaspoon pepper*

Brush chicken breasts lightly with olive oil and place in a baking pan which has been coated with olive oil cooking spray. Drizzle with lemon juice and sprinkle remaining ingredients evenly over chicken pieces.

Bake at 400° for 15 to 20 minutes or until tender and juices are clear. Broil for 1 minute to lightly brown chicken, if desired.

Serving size: 1 portion (1/6 recipe)
Analysis per serving: 102 Calories, 16 g Protein, tr Carbohydrate,
4 g Fat, 1 g Sat Fat, % Calories from Fat 31, 41 mg Cholesterol, 127 mg Sodium
Diabetic exchanges: 2 lean meats

Macaroni Turkey Salad

4 servings

1	cup shell-shaped macaroni
3	cups water
1	cup cubed cooked turkey breast
1	cup seedless grapes
1/4	cup sliced green onions

Dressing

2	tablespoons reduced-fat mayonnaise
2	tablespoons light sour cream
1	tablespoon cider vinegar
2	teaspoons Dijon mustard
1/2	teaspoon sugar
1/4	teaspoon white pepper
1/4	teaspoon dried dillweed

Cook macaroni in boiling water for 6 to 8 minutes. Drain in a colander, and rinse with cold water. Drain, cool and place in a medium bowl.

Add turkey, grapes and green onions to macaroni. Toss gently to combine. ☺

Mix dressing ingredients in a small bowl. Add to salad mixture and toss again to combine.

Cover and chill before serving.

Serving size: 1 cup
Analysis per serving: 215 Calories, 12 g Protein, 31 g Carbohydrate,
5 g Fat, 1 g Sat Fat, % Calories from Fat 21, 19 mg Cholesterol, 376 mg Sodium
Diabetic exchanges: 2 starches, 1 lean meat & 1/2 fat

ORIENTAL CHICKEN STIRFRY

6 servings

1	*pound boneless, skinless chicken breasts*
1	*tablespoon margarine*
1	*pound bag frozen mixed vegetables*
	(broccoli, carrots, and water chestnuts)
2	*tablespoons reduced-sodium soy sauce*
1/4	*teaspoon pepper*
2	*tablespoons diced pimento*
1	*tablespoon cornstarch*
1	*cup ready-to-serve chicken broth*

Cut chicken into 3/4-inch strips and set aside.

Melt margarine in a large nonstick skillet on medium heat. Add chicken; stirfry until it loses its pink color.

Add mixed vegetables, soy sauce, pepper and pimento.

In a separate bowl, combine cornstarch and chicken broth; stir well. Add broth mixture to chicken and vegetables, stirring until thickened.

Reduce heat to low; cover pan and simmer 5 minutes.

Serving size: 1 portion (1/6 recipe)
Analysis per serving: 171 Calories, 22 g Protein, 9 g Carbohydrate,
5 g Fat, 1 g Sat Fat, % Calories from Fat 25, 57 mg Cholesterol, 385 mg Sodium
Diabetic exchanges: 2 vegetables & 2 1/2 lean meats

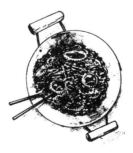

SKILLET CHICKEN & VEGETABLES

Serve with CELERY CABBAGE SALAD (page 124)
or COLESLAW (page 126).

6 servings

2	*teaspoons olive oil*
1	*pound boneless and skinless chicken breasts*
1	*pound small new potatoes, scrubbed*
1	*10-ounce package frozen sugar snap peas*
1/2	*cup water*
1/2	*teaspoon chicken-flavored bouillon granules*
2	*tablespoons dried minced onion*
1/4	*teaspoon garlic salt*
1/2	*teaspoon lemon pepper seasoning*

Heat olive oil in a large skillet over medium heat. Add chicken, and cook until lightly brown, turning as needed.

Place vegetables around chicken. Add all other ingredients. Cover and bring to a boil over medium heat. ☺

Reduce heat and simmer 25 minutes or until potatoes and chicken are tender.

Serving size: 1 chicken breast half and 1/6 vegetable mixture
Analysis per serving: 190 Calories, 19 g Protein, 19 g Carbohydrate,
4 g Fat, 1 g Sat Fat, % Calories from Fat 18, 41 mg Cholesterol, 230 mg Sodium
Diabetic exchanges: 1 starch, 1 vegetable & 2 lean meats

BEEF STEW

9 servings

1 1/2	pounds sirloin tip beef, cut for stew
1	14 1/2-ounce can stewed tomatoes with onion, pepper, and celery
1	8-ounce can tomato sauce
1	10 3/4-ounce can ready-to-serve beef broth
1	cup water
2	tablespoons Worcestershire sauce
1/4	teaspoon ground thyme
1/4	teaspoon marjoram
1/4	teaspoon pepper
1	24-ounce package frozen stew vegetables

Combine all ingredients except frozen vegetables, in a Dutch oven. Cover and bring to a boil; reduce heat and simmer 1 1/2 hours. ☺

Add vegetables, cover and cook an additional 30 minutes or until meat and vegetables are tender.

Serving size: 1 cup
Analysis per serving: 195 Calories, 22 g Protein, 17 g Carbohydrate,
4 g Fat, 1 g Sat Fat, % Calories from Fat 19, 49 mg Cholesterol, 450 mg Sodium
Diabetic exchanges: 1/2 starch, 2 vegetables & 2 lean meats

TURKEY SPINACH LASAGNA

If "no-boil" noodles are not available, use regular lasagna noodles.
Put the casserole together the day before and refrigerate
over-night, or let the noodles soften in cold water.
8 servings

Meat Sauce

3/4	*pound ground turkey*
1/2	*cup frozen chopped onion*
1	*cup fresh sliced mushrooms*
1	*14 1/2-ounce can Italian tomatoes*
1	*6-ounce can Italian tomato paste*
2	*tablespoons low-sodium Worcestershire sauce*
1	*cup water*
6	*ounces "no-boil" lasagna noodles*
1	*10-ounce box frozen chopped spinach, thawed*
1	*12-ounce carton low-fat cottage cheese*
1	*cup shredded part-skim Mozzarella cheese*
1/2	*cup fresh grated Parmesan cheese*

Combine turkey, onion, and mushrooms in a large non-stick skillet. Cook over low heat until meat is browned and vegetables are tender, stirring as needed to crumble meat. Add tomatoes, tomato paste, Worcestershire sauce and water, stir to mix. Simmer 15 minutes, stirring occasionally.☺

Spread about 1 1/4 cups of the meat sauce in a 9-x 13-x 2-inch pan. Place a layer of uncooked noodles over sauce. Spread about 1 1/4 cups of remaining sauce over noodle layer, then add layers of 1/2 the drained spinach, 1/2 the cottage cheese, and 1/2 of the mozzarella cheese.

Repeat layers of noodles, 1 1/4 cups meat sauce, remaining spinach, cottage cheese and mozzarella cheese. Cover with remaining noodles, then remaining sauce. Sprinkle Parmesan cheese over top.

Cover with foil and bake at 350° for 45 minutes. Uncover and cook an additional 10 minutes. Let stand 15 minutes before cutting into 8 equal portions to serve.

Serving size: 1 portion
Analysis per serving: 293 Calories, 24 g Protein, 29 g Carbohydrate,
9 g Fat, 4 g Sat Fat, % Calories from Fat 27, 38 mg Cholesterol, 522 mg Sodium
Diabetic exchanges: 1 1/2 starches, 1 1/2 vegetables & 2 medium-fat meats

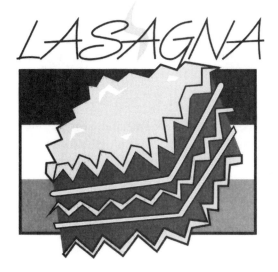

CHILI

This is a great recipe to freeze and reheat for later meals.
Try teaming it with CORNBREAD (page 193).
6 servings

1	*cup dried pinto beans*
3	*cups water*
1/2	*pound ground round*
1	*11 1/2-ounce can reduced-sodium vegetable tomato juice*
1-2	*teaspoons chili powder*
1/4	*teaspoon dried minced garlic*
1	*teaspoon dried minced onion*
1	*14 1/2-ounce can stewed tomatoes with onion and pepper*

Sort and rinse beans. Place water and beans in a Dutch oven. Soak overnight or boil two minutes; turn off heat and let stand 1 hour before cooking. Do not drain. Cover and bring to a boil; reduce heat and simmer 1 hour or until beans are tender. ☺

Cook meat in a nonstick skillet over medium heat, stirring to crumble meat. Add meat, vegetable tomato juice, seasonings and stewed tomatoes to beans in Dutch oven. Cover and bring to a boil; reduce heat, and simmer for 30 minutes, stirring as needed to prevent sticking.

Serving size: 1 cup
Analysis per serving: 170 Calories, 16 g Protein, 22 g Carbohydrate,
2 g Fat, 1 g Sat Fat, % Calories from Fat 13, 28 mg Cholesterol, 289 mg Sodium
Diabetic exchanges: 1 starch, 1 vegetable & 1 1/2 lean meats

HAMBURGER PIE

Using a pre-cooked pizza crust would reduce the calories and calories from fat in this recipe. Spread the cooked meat mixture then the cheese over the pizza crust, and heat in a 400° oven until cheese is melted.

6 servings

3/4	*pound ground round*
1/2	*cup chopped fresh or frozen onion*
3/4	*cup water*
1	*6-ounce can Italian-seasoned tomato paste*
1/2	*teaspoon garlic powder*
1	*prepared pie crust*
1/2	*cup shredded part-skim Mozzarella cheese*
1	*cup chopped lettuce*
1/4	*cup commercial picante sauce*

Place cookie sheet on rack in middle of oven set at 400° and preheat while making pie.

Cook ground round and onions in a large skillet over medium heat until meat is brown and onion is tender, stirring to crumble meat.

Add water, tomato paste, and garlic powder. Cover and bring to a boil; reduce heat and simmer for 10 minutes. ☺

Spoon meat mixture into an uncooked pie shell and bake for 15 to 20 minutes on preheated cookie sheet. Remove from oven and immediately top with grated cheese.

Cut into 6 servings. Just before serving, sprinkle 1 cup chopped lettuce evenly over pie. Top each serving with 2 teaspoons picante sauce.

Serving size: 1/6 pie
Analysis per serving: 295 Calories, 20 g Protein, 22 g Carbohydrate,
14 g Fat, 4 g Sat Fat, % Calories from Fat 42, 45 mg Cholesterol, 407 mg Sodium
Diabetic exchanges: 1 starch, 1 vegetable, 2 medium-fat meats & 1 fat

ITALIAN BEEF & PASTA

Freezes well!
6 servings

1/2	pound ground round
1/4	cup dried minced onion
1/2	teaspoon dried minced garlic
2	8-ounce cans no-salt-added tomato sauce
1	6-ounce can tomato paste
1	teaspoon dried Italian seasoning
2 1/2	cups water
1/2	teaspoon salt
1 1/2	cups uncooked corkscrew macaroni
1	cup shredded part-skim Mozzarella cheese

Cook ground round in a Dutch oven over low heat until meat is brown, stirring to crumble meat.

Add onion, garlic, tomato sauce, tomato paste, Italian seasoning, water and salt. Cover and bring to boil over medium heat; stirring occasionally to prevent sticking. ☺

Add pasta; cover and cook for 15 to 18 minutes or until pasta is done. Stir occasionally after adding pasta.

Remove from heat. Top with shredded cheese. Serve from Dutch oven.

Serving size: 1 cup
Analysis per serving: 276 Calories, 17 g Protein, 33 g Carbohydrate, ·
5 g Fat, 3 g Sat Fat, % Calories from Fat 18, 33 mg Cholesterol, 311 mg Sodium
Diabetic exchanges: 2 starches, 1 vegetable & 1 1/2 lean meats

POT ROAST

Ready-peeled small carrots are becoming widely available.
They are sometimes marketed as "baby" carrots.
6 servings

1	*tablespoon margarine*
2	*pounds eye of round roast*
1	*14 1/2-ounce can beef broth*
1	*cup water*
1/4	*teaspoon pepper*
1/4	*teaspoon garlic salt*
1	*pound new potatoes, unpeeled and scrubbed*
1	*pound ready-peeled small carrots*
2	*cups small, whole, frozen onions*

Heat margarine in a Dutch oven over medium heat until hot.

Add meat, and cook until evenly browned, turning as needed. ☺

Add broth, water, pepper, and garlic salt. Cover and bring to a boil. Reduce heat and simmer 1 1/2 hours. ☺

Place potatoes, carrots and onions around roast. Cover, return to a boil. Reduce heat and simmer an additional 45 minutes or until meat and vegetables are tender.

Transfer meat and vegetables to serving platter or serve directly from Dutch oven. Slice meat into 6 portions.

Serving size: 3 ounces meat with 1/6 vegetable mixture
Analysis per serving: 299 Calories, 28 g Protein, 26 g Carbohydrate,
9 g Fat, 3 g Sat Fat, % Calories from Fat 27, 60 mg Cholesterol, 401 mg Sodium
Diabetic exchanges: 1 1/2 starches, 1 vegetable & 3 lean meats

SAVORY BEEF
& NOODLE CASSEROLE

8 servings

3/4	*pound ground round*
1	*15-ounce can tomato sauce*
1/4	*teaspoon salt*
1/4	*teaspoon pepper*
1/4	*teaspoon dried minced garlic*
5	*green onions, chopped (including tops)*
4	*ounces light cream cheese*
8	*ounces fat-free sour cream*
1	*8-ounce package egg yolk-free noodles,*
	cooked according to package directions
Vegetable cooking spray	
1/2	*cup shredded reduced-fat sharp Cheddar cheese*

Cook ground round in a large nonstick skillet over medium heat until meat is brown, stirring to crumble meat.

Add tomato sauce, salt, pepper and garlic. Cover and simmer 15 minutes. ☺

In a small bowl, combine green onions, light cream cheese and sour cream.

Spread cooked, drained noodles in 9-x 12-inch baking dish coated with cooking spray. Spread ground meat mixture over noodles. Spread cream cheese mixture over ground beef. Sprinkle grated cheese over top.

Bake 15 to 20 minutes at 350°. Allow to cool 10 minutes before cutting into 8 portions.

Serving size: 1 portion
Analysis per serving: 266 Calories, 21 g Protein, 28 g Carbohydrate,
7 g Fat, 4 g Sat Fat, % Calories from Fat 24, 41 mg Cholesterol, 501 mg Sodium
Diabetic exchanges: 2 starches, 1/4 vegetable & 2 lean meats

TAMALE PIE

8 servings

1	*pound ground round*
1	*cup chopped fresh or frozen onion*
1	*14 1/2-ounce can Mexican stewed tomatoes*
1	*17-ounce can whole kernel corn, no salt added, drained*
1/2	*teaspoon salt*
1	*tablespoon chili powder*
1/2	*teaspoon ground cumin*
1/4	*teaspoon hot sauce*
1	*egg*
1	*cup self-rising cornmeal*
1	*cup skim milk*

Cook ground round and onion in a large skillet over medium heat until meat is brown and onion is tender, stirring to crumble meat.

Add tomatoes, corn, salt, chili powder, cumin and hot sauce. Cover, bring to a boil; reduce heat and simmer for 20 minutes. ☺

Spoon or pour into a 13-x 9-x 2-inch baking dish.

Mix egg, cornmeal, and skim milk in a small bowl. Pour cornmeal mixture over meat mixture. Bake for 30 minutes at 350° or until cornmeal is golden brown.

Serving size: 1 portion
Analysis per serving: 258 Calories, 17 g Protein, 32 g Carbohydrate,
7 g Fat, 3 g Sat Fat, % Calories from Fat 27, 58 mg Cholesterol, 512 mg Sodium
Diabetic exchanges: 2 starches, 1/4 vegetable & 1 1/2 medium-fat meats

HAM & POTATO CASSEROLE

Potatoes can be cooked, drained and held overnight in the refrigerator.
6 servings

2	*large potatoes, unpeeled and scrubbed*
4	*ounces (1 cup) chopped, cooked, lean ham*
1/2	*cup chopped fresh or frozen onion*
	Vegetable cooking spray

1	*cup skim milk*
2	*tablespoons flour*
1/4	*teaspoon paprika*
1/2	*cup shredded reduced-fat sharp Cheddar cheese*

Place potatoes in medium saucepan. Add water to 1 inch above potatoes and cover. Bring to a boil. Reduce heat and simmer 30 minutes or until potatoes are tender. ☺

Remove potatoes from water with a fork or slotted spoon. When cool enough to handle, cut potatoes into 1/2-inch slices.

Place potatoes, then ham and onion in a 2-quart casserole dish coated with cooking spray. ☺

Measure the milk in a 2 cup or larger measuring cup. Sprinkle flour and paprika over milk and use a whisk or hand-held mixer to blend.

Pour milk mixture over potatoes and ham. Top with cheese. Cover and bake at 350° for 30 minutes. Uncover and bake an additional 10 to 15 minutes.

Serving size: 1 portion
Analysis per serving: 179 Calories, 10 g Protein, 28 g Carbohydrate,
3 g Fat, 2 g Sat Fat, % Calories from Fat 15, 17 mg Cholesterol, 322 mg Sodium
Diabetic exchanges: 2 starches & 1/2 medium-fat meat

ROASTED PORK LOIN

12 servings

3	*pounds boneless pork loin roast*
2	*tablespoons soy sauce*
1	*tablespoon honey*
1/4	*teaspoon curry powder*

Place pork roast in a baking pan, insert meat thermometer. Bake uncovered for 1 hour at 325°.

Combine soy sauce, honey and curry powder in a small bowl. Spoon over surface of meat.

Continue cooking 30 minutes or until meat thermometer reaches 160° and juices are clear. Allow to cool for 10 minutes before slicing into 12 portions.

Serving size: 3 ounces
Analysis per serving: 177 Calories, 23 g Protein, 2 g Carbohydrate,
8 g Fat, 3 g Sat Fat, % Calories from Fat 41, 66 mg Cholesterol, 211 mg Sodium
Diabetic exchanges: 3 lean meats

SWEET & SOUR PORK

4 servings

Vegetable cooking spray
1   *pound boneless pork loin, well-trimmed and cut into strips*
1/4   *cup water*

1/4   *teaspoon salt*
2   *tablespoons sugar*
1   *tablespoon cornstarch*
1   *8-ounce can pineapple chunks, in its own juice*
1   *tablespoon low-sodium soy sauce*
1   *cup coarsely chopped green pepper*
1   *tablespoon cider vinegar*
2   *cups cooked egg yolk-free noodles (cooked without salt or fat)*

Spray nonstick skillet with cooking spray. Add pork strips and brown over medium heat, turning once, for approximately 5 minutes per side.

Add water to skillet; cover and cook over low heat for 15 minutes. ☺

Mix salt, sugar, cornstarch, pineapple and its juice, soy sauce, green pepper and vinegar in a small bowl.

Stir into pork and cook over medium heat 3 minutes or until thickened. Serve over 1/2 cup cooked noodles.

Serving size: 1/4 recipe
Analysis per serving: 392 Calories, 30 g Protein, 40 g Carbohydrate,
11 g Fat, 4 g Sat Fat, % Calories from Fat 25, 84 mg Cholesterol, 272 mg Sodium
Diabetic exchanges: 1 1/2 starches, 1 fruit, 1/2 vegetable & 3 1/2 medium-fat meats

Vegetables
&
Side Dishes

Contents

BROCCOLI WITH PIMENTO

3 servings

1	*10-ounce box frozen broccoli spears**
1/4	*teaspoon salt*
1	*tablespoon lemon juice*
2	*tablespoons chopped pimento*
1	*tablespoon sliced almonds*

Cook broccoli according to package directions, using 1/4 teaspoon salt. Remove broccoli from pan with a slotted spoon and place in a serving bowl.

Drizzle with lemon juice. Top with pimento and sliced almonds, and serve hot.

* French style or cut green beans may be substituted for broccoli.

Serving size: 1/3 of recipe
Analysis per serving: 39 Calories, 3 g Protein, 6 g Carbohydrate,
1 g Fat, tr Sat Fat, 0 mg Cholesterol, 190 mg Sodium
Diabetic exchange: 1 vegetable

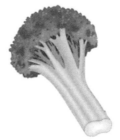

CHEESY BROCCOLI RICE CASSEROLE

This recipe can be made ahead, covered and refrigerated
in an oven-safe baking dish for reheating.
10 servings

1	*6.25-ounce package long grain and wild rice mixture (fast-cooking type)*
2	*cups water*
1	*tablespoon margarine*
1	*10-ounce package frozen chopped broccoli*
1/4	*cup frozen or fresh chopped onion*
1	*cup skim milk*
2	*tablespoons flour*
1/2	*cup shredded reduced-fat sharp Cheddar cheese*

Place uncooked rice, seasoning packet from rice, water, margarine, broccoli and onion in a medium saucepan. Cover and bring to a boil. Reduce heat to medium and cook for 6 minutes.☺

Measure milk in a large measuring cup. Sprinkle flour into cold milk and use mixer or whisk to blend. Add to cooked broccoli mixture and continue cooking on medium heat, stirring until mixture is thickened.

Remove from heat. Sprinkle cheese on top. Serve directly from the saucepan if desired.

For a baked casserole, place rice mixture in a 1 1/2-quart casserole dish, and bake at 350° for 10 minutes to melt cheese and set mixture.

Serving size: 1/2 cup
Analysis per serving: 110 Calories, 5 g Protein, 17 g Carbohydrate,
3 g Fat, 1 g Sat Fat, % Calories from Fat 20, 4 mg Cholesterol, 364 mg Sodium
Diabetic exchanges: 1 starch, 1/2 vegetable & 1/2 lean meat

GLAZED CARROTS

4 servings

2	teaspoons margarine
1	10-ounce box frozen sliced carrots
1/4	cup water
1/4	teaspoon chicken-flavored bouillon granules
2	tablespoons granulated brown sugar

Dash ground nutmeg

Melt margarine in a 1-quart saucepan over medium heat.

Add carrots, water, and chicken granules. Stir, cover and cook over medium heat for 10 to 12 minutes or until carrots are crisp-tender.

Add brown sugar and nutmeg. Increase heat and cook uncovered for approximately 2 minutes to reduce liquid. Stir as needed to prevent sticking.

Serving size: 1/2 cup
Analysis per serving: 70 Calories, 1 g Protein, 13 g Carbohydrate,
2 g Fat, tr Sat Fat, 0 mg Cholesterol, 118 mg Sodium
Diabetic exchanges: 1 vegetable & 1/2 starch

GREEN BEANS
WITH PEARL ONIONS

5 servings

1	10-ounce box frozen cut green beans
1	cup frozen whole pearl onions
1/4	teaspoon crushed marjoram
1	teaspoon margarine
1/4	teaspoon chicken-flavored bouillon granules
2	tablespoons water

Place all ingredients in a medium saucepan. Cover and bring to a boil. Reduce heat and simmer 10 minutes. Drain. Serve hot.

Serving size: 1/2 cups
Analysis per serving: 34 Calories, 1 g Protein, 6 g Carbohydrate,
1 g Fat, tr Sat Fat, 0 mg Cholesterol, 58 mg Sodium
Diabetic exchange: 1 vegetable

HOLIDAY PEAS
& CAULIFLOWER

8 servings

1	*10-ounce package frozen green peas*
1	*10-ounce package frozen cauliflower florets*
1/2	*cup chopped red pepper*
1/4	*teaspoon salt*
2	*teaspoons margarine*
1/2	*cup water*

Combine all ingredients in a 2-quart saucepan. Cover and bring to a boil. Reduce heat, and simmer for 8 to 10 minutes.

Transfer vegetables with a slotted spoon from pan to a serving dish. Serve hot.

Serving size: 1/2 cup
Analysis per serving: 44 Calories, 2 g Protein, 7 g Carbohydrate,
1 g Fat, tr Sat Fat, 0 mg Cholesterol, 109 mg Sodium
Diabetic exchanges: 1/2 vegetable & 1/2 starch

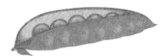

LEMON PEPPER SPINACH

3 servings

1	10-ounce box frozen spinach or 1 pound fresh spinach*
1	tablespoon lemon juice
1/4	teaspoon lemon pepper seasoning

Cook spinach according to package directions omitting salt. Drain.

Place in serving dish. Sprinkle lemon juice and lemon pepper seasoning over spinach. Toss lightly to mix. Serve hot.

* You can substitute zucchini or broccoli for spinach.

Serving size: 1/2 cup
Analysis per serving: 23 Calories, 2 g Protein, 4 g Carbohydrate,
tr g Fat, tr Sat Fat, 0 mg Cholesterol, 53 mg Sodium
Diabetic exchange: 1 vegetable

OVEN-BROWNED POTATOES

3 servings

1   16-ounce can small white potatoes, drained
Olive oil cooking spray
Dash garlic powder
1   teaspoon dried parsley
Dash pepper
1/4   teaspoon dried Italian seasoning
1   tablespoon grated Parmesan cheese

Place potatoes in a 1-quart baking dish which has been coated with cooking spray. Sprinkle remaining ingredients evenly over potatoes. Bake at 400° for 30 minutes or until lightly browned.

Serving size: 1/3 of recipe
Analysis per serving: 50 Calories, 2 g Protein, 10 g Carbohydrate,
1 g Fat, tr Sat Fat, 1 mg Cholesterol, 308 mg Sodium
Diabetic exchange: 1/2 starch

POTATOES SUPREME

Can be made ahead and refrigerated, covered, until ready to reheat.
Store foods that are difficult to pour (like instant potatoes)
in airtight containers from which you can dip the needed amount.
6 servings

1 1/2	*cups hot water*
1/2	*teaspoon salt*
1	*cup skim milk*
2	*cups instant potatoes*
1/2	*cup plain nonfat yogurt*
4	*fresh chopped green onions (including tops)*
1/2	*cup shredded reduced-fat sharp Cheddar cheese*

Bring water to boil and remove from heat. Add salt and skim milk. Stir in instant potatoes until smooth.

Combine potatoes, yogurt and green onions. Place potato mixture in a 1-quart casserole dish. Top with grated cheese. Heat in 350° oven about 20 minutes or until hot.

Serving size: 1/2 cup
Analysis per serving: 111 Calories, 7 g Protein, 17 g Carbohydrate,
2 g Fat, 1 g Sat Fat, % Calories from Fat 15, 6 mg Cholesterol, 276 mg Sodium
Diabetic exchanges: 1/2 starch, 1/2 skim milk & 1/2 fat

POTLUCK HASHBROWN CASSEROLE

8 servings

1	1 pound, 10-ounce bag hash brown potatoes
1/2	cup onion, frozen and chopped
1	cup shredded, reduced-fat Cheddar cheese
3/4	cup fat-free sour cream
1	10 1/2-ounce can 99% fat-free cream of chicken soup
1/2	teaspoon salt

Vegetable cooking spray
1   *tablespoon toasted bread crumbs*

Stir together first 6 ingredients and place in a 1 1/2 quart baking dish which has been coated with vegetable cooking spray.

Sprinkle bread crumbs over top. Bake at 350° for 1 1/4 hours or until potatoes are tender.

Serving size: 1/2 cup
Analysis per serving: 167 Calories, 8 g Protein, 26 g Carbohydrate,
3 g Fat, 2 g Sat Fat, % Calories from Fat 18, 10 mg Cholesterol, 385 mg Sodium
Diabetic exchanges: 2 starches & 1/2 fat

SPICED SWEET POTATOES WITH APPLES

Sweet potatoes may be prepared in advance
and chilled overnight for ease in handling.
6 servings

2	*medium sweet potatoes*
1	*cup unsweetened canned apple slices*
1	*tablespoon margarine* → ½ TB/OLIVE OIL
1/4	*cup granulated brown sugar* → ¼ C SPLENDA
1/4	*teaspoon pumpkin pie spice* ½ Tsp

Place sweet potatoes in a Dutch oven. Add water to 1 inch above potatoes, and cover. Bring to a boil, reduce heat and simmer for 35 minutes or until potatoes are tender.☺

Remove sweet potatoes from water with a fork or slotted spoon and let cool; peel and cut into bite-size pieces.

Place potatoes and remaining ingredients in a large nonstick skillet; stir gently to combine. Cook mixture over medium heat for 5 minutes or until thoroughly heated, stirring as needed to prevent sticking.

Serving size: 1/2 cup
Analysis per serving: 137 Calories, 1 g Protein, 30 g Carbohydrate,
2 g Fat, tr Sat Fat, % Calories from Fat 13, 0 mg Cholesterol, 33 mg Sodium
Diabetic exchanges: 1 starch, 1 fruit & 1/2 fat

SQUASH CASSEROLE

4 servings

3/4	*pound yellow squash*
1/2	*cup chopped fresh or frozen onion*
1/4	*teaspoon salt*

Dash pepper

2	*tablespoons water*

1/4	*cup cracker crumbs*
1	*egg white, stirred with a fork*
1/4	*cup skim milk*
1/4	*cup shredded sharp reduced-fat Cheddar cheese, divided*

Vegetable cooking spray

Wash and cut squash into 1/4-inch slices.

Combine squash, onion, salt, pepper and water in a saucepan. Cover and bring to a boil. Reduce heat to medium and cook for 20 minutes. ☺

Remove squash from heat, and mash the mixture with a vegetable masher.

Add cracker crumbs, egg, milk, and half the cheese to squash. Mix well.

Pour or spoon squash mixture into a baking dish pan coated with cooking spray. Top with remaining cheese. Bake uncovered at 350° for 20 minutes or until cheese is melted, but not browned, and mixture is set.

Serving size: 1/2 cup
Analysis per serving: 63 Calories, 4 g Protein, 8 g Carbohydrate,
2 g Fat, 1 g Sat Fat, 4 mg Cholesterol, 227 mg Sodium
Diabetic exchanges: 1 1/2 vegetables & 1/4 medium-fat meat

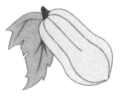

STEAMED FRESH VEGETABLES

If your store's produce section does not have ready-peeled
baby carrots, use 4 peeled regular carrots.

4 servings

1/4	*pound whole green beans, with ends and strings removed*
1/2	*medium head cabbage, cut into 4 wedges*
16	*ready-peeled baby carrots*
4	*small new potatoes, scrubbed and unpeeled*
4	*small summer squash, cut into halves*
3/4	*cup water*
1	*tablespoon margarine*
1	*teaspoon dried dillweed*
1/4	*teaspoon salt*

Place all vegetables in Dutch oven. Add water. Cover and bring water to a
boil. Reduce heat and simmer vegetables for 20 minutes or until tender.

Remove from pan with a slotted spoon to a serving dish.

Melt margarine in a small saucepan. Add dillweed and salt; stir to combine.
Drizzle over cooked vegetables.

Serving size: 1/4 recipe
Analysis per serving: 156 Calories, 4 g Protein, 29 g Carbohydrate,
4 g Fat, tr Sat Fat, 0 mg Cholesterol, 163 mg Sodium
Diabetic exchanges: 1 starch, 2 vegetables & 1 fat

TOMATOES & OKRA

Zucchini may be substituted for okra.
6 servings

1	*teaspoon olive oil*
1/2	*cup frozen chopped onion*
1	*10-ounce package frozen okra*
1	*14 1/2-ounce can Italian-seasoned tomatoes*

Dash pepper

Heat oil over medium heat in a 2-quart nonstick saucepan. Add onion; cook for 2 minutes, or until transparent, over medium heat.

Add remaining ingredients; stir to combine. Reduce heat, cover and simmer for 10 minutes, stirring occasionally.

Serving size: 1/2 cup
Analysis per serving: 41 Calories, 2 g Protein, 7 g Carbohydrate,
1 g Fat, tr Sat Fat, 0 mg Cholesterol, 226 mg Sodium
Diabetic exchange: 1 vegetable

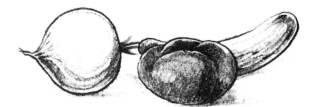

ZUCCHINI PARMESAN

6 servings

1	*pound zucchini, washed and cut into 1/4 inch slices*
2	*tablespoons water*
1/4	*teaspoon salt*

Dash pepper

1/4	*cup fresh grated Parmesan cheese*

Place zucchini in large nonstick skillet. Add water, salt and pepper. Cook over medium heat until hot. Reduce heat, cover and simmer for 10 minutes or until zucchini is crisp tender.

Sprinkle cheese over top and cook until cheese is melted (about 2 minutes) without stirring. Serve directly from pan if desired.

Serving size: 1/2 cup
Analysis per serving: 35 Calories, 3 g Protein, 3 g Carbohydrate,
1 g Fat, 1 g Sat Fat, 3 mg Cholesterol, 166 mg Sodium
Diabetic exchange: 1 vegetable

BLACK-EYED PEAS & RICE
(Hoppinjohn)

4 servings

Vegetable cooking spray
1   cup frozen chopped onion
1/2   cup fresh or frozen chopped green pepper
1   15-ounce can black-eyed peas, drained
1/8   teaspoon dried minced garlic
1/4   teaspoon red pepper flakes
1/4   teaspoon thyme
2   cups cooked rice (cooked without salt or fat)

Coat a 2-quart saucepan with cooking spray and place over medium heat. Add onion and green pepper and cook, stirring occasionally, for 5 minutes or until vegetables are tender.

Add remaining ingredients (except rice), stirring to blend. Cover and simmer 15 minutes. Serve over hot rice.

Serving size: 1/2 cup black-eyed pea mixture and 1/2 cup rice
Analysis per serving: 215 Calories, 11 g Protein, 41 g Carbohydrate,
1 g Fat, tr Sat Fat, % Calories from Fat 5, 0 mg Cholesterol, 257 mg Sodium
Diabetic exchanges: 2 1/2 starches & 1/2 vegetable

BULGUR PILAF

You can substitute rice or couscous for bulgur.
8 servings

2	*cups pre-sliced fresh mushrooms*
1	*cup bulgur*
2	*cups ready-to-serve chicken broth*
2	*teaspoons dried minced onion*
1/4	*teaspoon salt*

Place all ingredients in a 2-quart saucepan. Cover and bring to a boil. Reduce heat and simmer 15 minutes or until liquid is absorbed.

Serving size: 1/2 cup
Analysis per serving: 110 Calories, 3 g Protein, 24 g Carbohydrate,
1 g Fat, tr Sat Fat, % Calories from Fat 6, 0 mg Cholesterol, 248 mg Sodium
Diabetic exchanges: 1 1/2 starches

LENTILS

5 servings

1	cup dried lentils
2 1/2	cups water
1	cup frozen mixed celery, pepper and onions
1/4	teaspoon minced dried garlic

Dash pepper

1/2	teaspoon salt
1	bay leaf

Place all ingredients in a large saucepan. Cover, bring to a boil, reduce heat and simmer for 1 1/4 hours. ☺

Remove bay leaf before serving.

Serving size: 1/2 cup
Analysis per serving: 141 Calories, 11 g Protein, 24 g Carbohydrate,
tr Fat, tr Sat Fat, % Calories from Fat 3, 0 mg Cholesterol, 206 mg Sodium
Diabetic exchanges: 1 1/2 starches & 1 lean meat

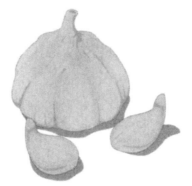

Breads

Contents

BANANA NUT BREAD

16 servings

3	*medium-sized ripe bananas*
1	*egg*
2	*cups all-purpose flour*
3/4	*cup sugar*
1/4	*teaspoon salt*
1	*teaspoon baking soda*
1/4	*cup chopped pecans*

Vegetable cooking spray

Preheat oven to 350°. Place bananas in medium mixing bowl and beat until smooth. Add egg and beat until light in color.

In a separate bowl, combine flour, sugar, salt, baking soda, and pecans. Add dry ingredients to banana mixture and mix until dry ingredients are moistened.

Spoon or pour batter into an 8 1/2-x 4 1/2-x 3-inch loafpan coated with cooking spray. Bake for 45 to50 minutes or until a wooden pick inserted in center comes out clean.

Cool bread in pan 10 minutes. Remove from pan, and cool completely on a wire rack. Cut bread into 16 slices.

Serving size: 1 slice
Analysis per serving: 122 Calories, 2 g Protein, 25 g Carbohydrate,
2 g Fat, tr Sat Fat, 16 mg Cholesterol, 86 mg Sodium
Diabetic exchanges: 1 starch, 3/4 fruit & 1/2 fat

BATTER BREAD

20 servings

2   tablespoons margarine
1   cup skim milk
1   cup water

4   cups all-purpose flour
4   tablespoons sugar
1   teaspoon salt
2   packages rapid rise yeast
Vegetable cooking spray

Melt margarine in a small saucepan over medium heat. Add milk and water to saucepan and heat until warm (105° to 115°). Remove from heat.

Place flour, sugar, salt, and yeast in a large mixer bowl. Attach dough hook to mixer and start mixer on low speed. Slowly pour milk mixture into dry ingredients while mixing. Mix at medium speed 2 to 3 minutes.

Raise dough hook out of bowl and let dough rise in place in mixer bowl for 45 minutes. ☺

Lower dough hook into batter and beat for 2 to 3 minutes.

Pour batter into a 10-inch tube pan coated with cooking spray. Bake at 375° for 35 minutes or until bread sounds hollow when thumped with finger.

Remove immediately from the pan and cool on a wire rack. Cut bread into 20 slices.

Serving size: 1 slice
Analysis per serving: 104 Calories, 3 g Protein, 20 g Carbohydrate,
2 g Fat, tr Sat Fat, tr Cholesterol, 119 mg Sodium
Diabetic exchanges: 1 1/4 starches & 1/2 fat

CORNBREAD

12 servings

1 1/2	*cups self-rising cornmeal*
1/2	*cup all-purpose flour*
1	*teaspoon sugar*
1	*egg*
1	*cup skim milk*
2	*tablespoons vegetable oil*
Vegetable cooking spray	

Preheat oven to 425°. Place all ingredients in a medium bowl; stir to mix well.

Pour into a 9-inch square baking pan which has been coated with cooking spray. Bake for 25 minutes or until lightly browned.

Cut into 12 portions, and serve hot.

Serving size: 1 square
Analysis per serving: 111 Calories, 3 g Protein, 17 g Carbohydrate,
4 g Fat, 1 g Sat Fat, 22 mg Cholesterol, 247 mg Sodium
Diabetic exchanges: 1 starch & 1 fat

ORANGE WHOLE WHEAT QUICK BREAD

16 servings

1 1/2   cups self-rising flour
1 1/2   cups whole wheat flour
1/4   teaspoon soda
3/4   cup sugar

3/4   cup orange juice
1/4   cup vegetable oil
1/2   cup skim milk
1   egg
1/2   teaspoon dried minced orange peel
Vegetable cooking spray

Topping
1   teaspoon sugar
1/2   teaspoon ground cinnamon

Preheat oven to 350°. Combine first 4 ingredients in a large bowl and set aside.

Stir together orange juice, oil, milk, egg and orange peel. Combine orange juice mixture with dry ingredients; stirring just until dry ingredients are moistened.

Pour into an 8 1/2 x 4 1/2 x 3-inch loafpan coated with cooking spray. Combine topping ingredients in a small bowl and sprinkle over top of batter.

Bake for 45 minutes or until wooden pick inserted in center comes out clean. Remove from pan immediately and cool completely on a wire rack.

Cut bread into 16 slices.

Measuring Hint: Measuring and mixing the liquid ingredients in a 2 cup measuring cup is a snap. Begin with 3/4 cup orange juice; add oil to the 1 cup mark; milk to 1 1/2 cup mark, then add egg and orange peel and combine with a wire whisk or hand-held mixer.

Serving size: 1 slice
Analysis per serving: 162 Calories, 3 g Protein, 29 g Carbohydrate,
4 g Fat, 1 g Sat Fat, 17 mg Cholesterol, 142 mg Sodium
Diabetic exchanges: 1 starch, 1 fruit & 1 fat

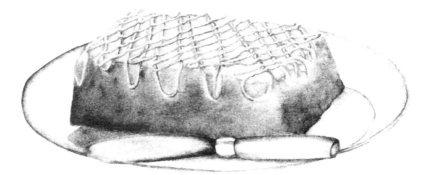

PECAN BREAKFAST BREAD

Granulated brown sugar is a pourable form of brown sugar
which is easily measured. No packing is necessary.
It is found by the regular sugars in supermarkets.
16 servings

3	*cups self-rising flour*
1	*teaspoon ground cinnamon*
1	*cup granulated brown sugar*
1 3/4	*cups skim milk*
2	*tablespoons vegetable oil*
1/3	*cup chopped pecans*

Vegetable cooking spray

Preheat oven to 325°. Combine flour, cinnamon and brown sugar in a large bowl. Add milk, oil and pecans, stirring until well blended.

Pour into an 8 1/2 x 4 1/2 x 3-inch loafpan coated with cooking spray. Bake 50 minutes or until toothpick inserted in center comes out clean. Cool bread in pan 10 minutes. Remove from pan and cool completely on a wire rack. Cut bread into 16 slices.

Serving size: 1 slice
Analysis per serving: 168 Calories, 3 g Protein, 31 g Carbohydrate,
4 g Fat, 1 g Sat Fat, 1 mg Cholesterol, 249 mg Sodium
Diabetic exchanges: 1 starch, 1 fruit & 1 fat

PRUNE PUMPKIN BREAD

2 loaves (16 servings each)

1 1/3	cups (8 ounces) pitted prunes
3/4	cup water
1	cup granulated brown sugar
1	cup sugar
2	eggs
1	cup pumpkin (about 1/2 of 16-ounce can)
2 1/2	cups self-rising flour
1	teaspoon baking soda
1	teaspoon cinnamon
1/4	teaspoon ground cloves
1/4	teaspoon ground ginger
	Vegetable cooking spray

Preheat oven to 350°. Combine prunes and water in blender or food processor container. Process until prunes are finely chopped. Stir together prune mixture, sugars, eggs and pumpkin in a large bowl. Set aside.

Combine flour, soda, cinnamon, cloves and ginger. Stir dry ingredients thoroughly.

Combine two mixtures with a spoon just until dry ingredients are moistened.

Coat two 8 1/2 x 4 1/2-inch loaf pans with vegetable cooking spray. Spoon mixture into pans, dividing equally. Bake 50 to 60 minutes or until pick inserted into centers comes out clean.

Remove from pan. Allow to cook completely on a wire rack. Cut each loaf into 16 slices.

Serving size: 1 slice
Analysis per serving: 110 Calories, 2 g Protein, 25 g Carbohydrate,
tr Fat, tr Sat Fat, 13 mg Cholesterol, 135 mg Sodium
Diabetic exchanges: 1 starch & 3/4 fruit

PUMPKIN DATE BREAD

This recipe makes 2 loaves — one for you and one for a gift!
Cover with plastic wrap and add a bow.
2 loaves (16 servings each)

1	*16-ounce can pumpkin*
2	*eggs*
1/2	*cup vegetable oil*
1 1/2	*cups granulated brown sugar*
1	*6-ounce can frozen apple juice concentrate, thawed and undiluted*
2	*teaspoons pumpkin pie spice*
1/2	*teaspoon baking soda*
4	*cups self-rising flour*
1	*cup chopped dates*
	Vegetable cooking spray

Preheat oven to 350°. In a large bowl combine pumpkin, eggs, oil, brown sugar, and apple juice. Set aside.

In a separate bowl combine spice, soda, flour and dates. Add flour mixture to pumpkin mixture; stir to combine just until dry ingredients are moistened.

Pour into two 8 1/2 x 4 1/2 x 3-inch loaf pans coated with cooking spray. Bake for 1 hour or until wooden pick inserted in center comes out clean.

Cool bread in pan for 10 minutes. Remove from pan and cool completely on a wire rack. Cut each loaf into 16 slices.

Variation: Raisins may be used instead of dates.

Serving size: 1 slice
Analysis per serving: 159 Calories, 2 g Protein, 29 Carbohydrate,
4 g Fat, 1 g Sat Fat, 16 mg Cholesterol, 183 mg Sodium
Diabetic exchanges: 1 starch, 1 fruit & 1 fat

WHOLE WHEAT BANANA BREAD

16 servings

3	medium-sized ripe bananas
1	egg
1	cup all-purpose flour
1	cup whole wheat flour
3/4	cup sugar
1/4	teaspoon salt
1	teaspoon baking soda
Vegetable cooking spray	

Preheat oven to 350°. Place bananas in a medium mixing bowl and beat until smooth. Add egg and beat until light in color. Set aside.

Stir together flours, sugar, salt and baking soda. Add dry ingredients to banana mixture. Stir until dry ingredients are moistened.

Spoon or pour batter into an 8 1/2- x 4 1/2- x 3-inch loaf pan coated with cooking spray. Bake for 45 to 50 minutes or until a wooden pick inserted in center comes out clean.

Remove from pan, and cool completely on a wire rack. Cut bread into 16 slices.

Serving size: 1 slice
Analysis per serving: 113 Calories, 2 g Protein, 26 Carbohydrate,
1 g Fat, tr Sat Fat, 16 mg Cholesterol, 86 mg Sodium
Diabetic exchanges: 1 starch & 3/4 fruit

HOLIDAY PINEAPPLE DATE MUFFINS

1 dozen muffins

4	*tablespoons margarine*
1/3	*cup sugar*
1	*egg*
1	*8-ounce can crushed unsweetened pineapple*
2	*cups self-rising flour*
1/2	*cup pitted, chopped dates*
1/4	*cup sliced maraschino cherries, well-drained*

Vegetable cooking spray

Preheat oven to 375°. Combine margarine, sugar and egg in a medium bowl; beat at medium speed of an electric mixer 2 minutes until light in color.

Add pineapple and flour; mix well. Stir in dates and cherries.

Spoon into 12 muffin cups which have been coated with cooking spray. Bake for about 25 minutes or until golden brown.

Serving size: 1 muffin
Analysis per serving: 168 Calories, 3 g Protein, 27 g Carbohydrate,
5 g Fat, 1 g Sat Fat, 22 mg Cholesterol, 258 mg Sodium
Diabetic exchanges: 1 starch, 1 fruit & 1 fat

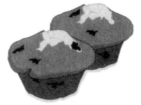

LEMON YOGURT MUFFINS

1 dozen muffins

2	cups self-rising flour
1/2	teaspoon baking soda
1/3	cup sugar
1	egg
1	8-ounce carton low-fat lemon yogurt*
1	tablespoon lemon juice
3	tablespoons vegetable oil

Vegetable cooking spray

Preheat oven to 375°. Combine flour and soda by stirring together in a large bowl; make a well in center of mixture. Set aside.

Combine remaining ingredients in a small bowl. Pour the liquid mixture into the well; stir just until dry ingredients are moistened.

Spoon mixture evenly into 12 muffin cups coated with cooking spray, filling two-thirds full. Bake for 15 to 20 minutes or until lightly browned.

Remove from pan and cool on a wire rack.

*Custard-type yogurt is not suitable for this recipe.

Serving size: 1 muffin
Analysis per serving: 148 Calories, 3 g Protein, 25 g Carbohydrate,
3 g Fat, 1 g Sat Fat, 19 mg Cholesterol, 357 mg Sodium
Diabetic exchanges: 1 starch, 1/2 fruit & 1/2 fat

PUMPKIN BRAN MUFFINS

1 dozen muffins

1 1/2	cups self-rising flour
1/2	cup sugar
1/2	teaspoon baking soda
1	teaspoon cinnamon
1	egg
1	cup canned pumpkin
1	cup flaked bran cereal
3/4	cup skim milk
1/2	cup light corn syrup

Vegetable cooking spray

Preheat oven to 400°. Combine flour, sugar, baking soda and cinnamon in a medium bowl and set aside.

Using a fork or wire whisk, beat egg lightly in a separate bowl. Stir in pumpkin, cereal, milk, and corn syrup. Add flour mixture and stir until well blended.

Spoon evenly into 12 muffin cups coated with vegetable cooking spray. Bake 18 to 20 minutes or until lightly browned and firm to the touch. Remove from pan and cool on a wire rack.

Serving size: 1 muffin
Analysis per serving: 157 Calories, 3 g Protein, 36 g Carbohydrate,
1 g Fat, 0 g Sat Fat, 18 mg Cholesterol, 300 mg Sodium
Diabetic exchanges: 1 starch & 1 1/2 fruits

RAISIN BRAN MUFFINS

Refrigerated batter will keep for 2 weeks.
Paper liners can be used to minimize work in cleaning the muffin pan.
1 dozen muffins

1	cup flaked bran cereal
1	teaspoon pumpkin pie spice
1/3	cup granulated brown sugar
1	cup skim milk
1	egg
3	tablespoons vegetable oil
1/2	cup raisins
1	teaspoon vanilla extract
1 3/4	cups self-rising flour
	Vegetable cooking spray

Preheat oven to 350°. Combine cereal, pumpkin pie spice, brown sugar and milk in a large bowl. Let stand for 2 minutes to soften cereal.

Stir in egg, oil, raisins and vanilla. Add flour; stir just until flour is moistened.

Spoon batter evenly into 12 muffin cups coated with cooking spray. Bake for 22 to 25 minutes or until lightly browned. Remove from pan and cool on a wire rack.

Serving size: 1 muffin
Analysis per serving: 160 Calories, 3 g Protein, 28 g Carbohydrate,
4 g Fat, 1 g Sat Fat, 22 mg Cholesterol, 234 mg Sodium
Diabetic exchanges: 1 starch, 1 fruit & 1 fat

SWEET POTATO MUFFINS

1 dozen muffins

4	*tablespoons margarine, softened*
3/4	*cup sugar*
1	*egg*
2/3	*cup canned sweet potatoes, drained*
1/4	*cup skim milk*
1	*cup flour*
1/4	*teaspoon salt*
1/4	*teaspoon ground cinnamon*
1/2	*teaspoon baking soda*

Vegetable cooking spray

Preheat oven to 375°. Cream margarine and sugar at medium speed with an electric mixer until light and fluffy. Add egg, sweet potatoes and skim milk. Blend well and set aside.

Stir dry ingredients together in a small bowl. Stir flour mixture into sweet potato mixture just until dry ingredients are moistened.

Spoon batter evenly into muffin pans coated with cooking spray. Bake for 25 minutes or until lightly browned. Remove from pan and cool on a wire rack.

Serving size: 1 muffin
Analysis per serving: 145 Calories, 2 g Protein, 24 g Carbohydrate,
5 g Fat, 1 g Sat Fat, 22 mg Cholesterol, 133 mg Sodium
Diabetic exchanges: 1 1/2 starches & 1 fat

CINNAMON COFFEE CAKE

Coffee cake may be baked at time of preparation
or refrigerated overnight and baked the next day.
May be frozen after baking.
15 servings

1/3	cup vegetable oil
1/2	cup sugar
1/2	cup granulated brown sugar
1	egg
2	cups self-rising flour
1	cup skim buttermilk
2	tablespoons nonfat dry powdered milk
1/2	teaspoon baking soda
1	teaspoon ground cinnamon

Vegetable cooking spray

Topping

1/3	cup granulated brown sugar
1/2	teaspoon ground cinnamon
2	tablespoons chopped pecans

Preheat oven to 350°. Combine ingredients in order given using an electric mixer on medium speed.

Spoon or pour batter into a 13-x 9-x 2-inch baking pan coated with cooking spray. Mix topping ingredients in a small bowl and sprinkle topping over batter. Bake for 30 minutes or until a wooden pick inserted in center comes out clean.

Cool completely in pan and cut into 15 portions and serve from pan.

Serving size: 1 portion
Analysis per serving: 189 Calories, 3 g Protein, 31 g Carbohydrate,
6 g Fat, 1 g Sat Fat, 18 mg Cholesterol, 220 mg Sodium
Diabetic exchanges: 2 starches & 1 fat

DROP BISCUITS

1 dozen biscuits

2   cups self-rising flour
3   tablespoons vegetable oil
1   cup nonfat buttermilk
Vegetable cooking spray

Preheat oven to 425°. Combine flour, oil and buttermilk in a medium bowl, stirring until well mixed.

Drop by spoonfuls onto baking sheet lightly coated with cooking spray. Bake for 8 to 10 minutes or until lightly browned.

Variation: 1/4 cup grated reduced-fat Cheddar cheese may be added. Cheese would increase fat and sodium.

Serving size: 1 biscuit
Analysis per serving: 106 Calories, 2 g Protein, 15 g Carbohydrate,
4 g Fat, 1 g Sat Fat, 1 mg Cholesterol, 280 mg Sodium
Diabetic exchanges: 1 starch & 1 fat

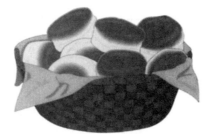

WHOLE WHEAT ROLLS

1 dozen rolls

1 1/2   cups all-purpose flour
1 1/2   cups whole wheat flour
1/3   cup sugar
1   teaspoon salt
2   packages rapid rise yeast

4   tablespoons margarine
1 1/2   cups skim milk
Vegetable cooking spray

Preheat oven to 400°. Put flours, sugar, salt and yeast in mixer bowl; stir with spoon.

Heat margarine and milk in a saucepan until warm, 105° to 115°. Remove from heat.

Attach dough hook to mixer and start mixer on low. Slowly pour warm milk mixture into dry ingredients while mixing. Mix at medium speed 2 to 3 minutes.

Raise dough hook out of bowl and let dough rise in mixing bowl for about 30 minutes. ☺

Lower dough hook back down into batter and beat for 2 to 3 minutes.

Spoon batter evenly into muffin pan coated with cooking spray. Bake for 25 minutes or until browned. Remove from the pan and serve warm.

Serving size: 1 roll
Analysis per serving: 175 Calories, 5 g Protein, 29 g Carbohydrate,
5 g Fat, 1 g Sat Fat, 1 mg Cholesterol, 226 mg Sodium
Diabetic exchanges: 2 starches & 1 fat

Desserts

Contents

VANILLA CUSTARD SAUCE

10 servings

1	*cup skim milk*
1	*egg yolk*
1	*tablespoon cornstarch*
3	*tablespoons sugar*
1/2	*teaspoon vanilla extract*

Dash nutmeg

Combine milk and egg yolk in a small bowl. Set aside.

Combine cornstarch and sugar in a small nonstick saucepan. Blend in milk mixture with a wire whisk or hand-held mixer.

Cook over medium heat, stirring constantly, until thickened. Remove from heat and stir in vanilla and nutmeg.

Serve with bread pudding or on plain cake or fruit for dessert.

Serving size: 2 tablespoons
Analysis per serving: 32 Calories, 1 g Protein, 6 g Carbohydrate,
1 g Fat, tr Sat Fat, 28 mg Cholesterol, 14 mg Sodium
Diabetic exchange: 1/2 starch

CHOCOLATE POUND CAKE

24 servings

1/2	cup (1 stick) margarine, softened
1 1/2	cups sugar
1	8-ounce carton egg substitute
3	cups flour
1/2	cup cocoa
1	teaspoon baking powder
1/4	teaspoon salt
1	cup skim milk
2	teaspoons vanilla
1/2	cup light corn syrup
Vegetable cooking spray	

Preheat over to 375°. Cream margarine and sugar in a large bowl, beating at medium speed of electric mixer until light and fluffy (about 5 minutes). Add egg substitute and beat until blended.

Stir together flour, cocoa, baking powder and salt in a separate bowl. Add to creamed mixture alternately with milk, beginning and ending with flour mixture. Mix just until blended after each addition. Blend in vanilla and corn syrup.☺

Pour batter into a 10-inch Bundt or tube pan coated with cooking spray.

Bake for 45 minutes or until a wooden pick inserted in center comes out clean.

Let stand for 10 minutes before removing from pan to cool on a wire rack. Allow to cool completely before cutting into 24 slices.

Serving size: 1 slice
Analysis per serving: 173 Calories, 3 g Protein, 30 g Carbohydrate,
4 g Fat, 1 g Sat Fat, tr Cholesterol, 123 mg Sodium
Diabetic exchanges: 2 starches & 1 fat

ORANGE POUND CAKE

24 servings

1 1/2	cups sugar
1/2	cup (1 stick) margarine, softened
2	eggs
2	egg whites
2 1/2	cups flour
2	teaspoons baking powder
1/2	cup skim milk
1/2	cup orange juice
Vegetable cooking spray	

Glaze
1/2	cup sugar
1/4	cup orange juice

Preheat over to 375º. Cream sugar and margarine in a large bowl, beating at medium speed of electric mixer until light and fluffy (about 5 minutes). Add eggs and egg whites and beat until well mixed.

Stir together flour and baking powder. Add to creamed mixture alternately with milk and orange juice, beginning and ending with flour mixture. Mix just until blended after each addition. ☺

Pour or spoon batter into a 10-inch tube pan coated with cooking spray.

Bake for 45 minutes or until wooden pick inserted in the center comes out clean.

Combine sugar and orange juice in a small pan. Cook over medium heat, stirring until sugar dissolves. Pour warm glaze over hot cake in pan. Allow cake to cool in pan 10 minutes. Move to a serving plate to cool completely. Cut cake into 24 slices.

Serving size: 1 slice
Analysis per serving: 155 Calories, 2 g Protein, 27 g Carbohydrate,
5 g Fat, 1 g Sat Fat, 22 mg Cholesterol, 95 mg Sodium
Diabetic exchanges: 1 starch, 3/4 fruit & 1 fat

FROZEN LEMON CHIFFON DESSERT

9 squares

1	*cup graham cracker crumbs*
1	*12-ounce can evaporated skim milk*
1/2	*cup fresh or bottled lemon juice*
1	*cup sugar*
1 or 2	*drops yellow food coloring*

Spread graham cracker crumbs in a 9-inch square pan and set aside.

Chill evaporated skim milk several hours or overnight. Pour chilled milk into a large bowl; beat at high speed of an electric mixer until stiff. Add lemon juice and sugar; mix well.

Spoon or pour onto the graham cracker crumbs. Freeze. Remove from the freezer about half an hour before serving to allow to soften before cutting into 9 portions. Serve immediately.

Serving size: 1 square
Analysis per serving: 158 Calories, 4 g Protein, 35 g Carbohydrate,
1 g Fat, tr Sat Fat, 2 mg Cholesterol, 115 mg Sodium
Diabetic exchanges: 1 1/4 starches & 1 fruit

PEACH COBBLER

9 servings

1   *tablespoon cornstarch*
1/3   *cup sugar*
2   *16-ounce cans sliced peaches in extra light syrup, undrained*
Dash nutmeg
1/4   *teaspoon almond extract*
Vegetable cooking spray

Topping
3   *tablespoons margarine, melted*
1/3   *cup sugar*
1   *cup self-rising flour*
1/3   *cup skim milk*

Preheat oven to 400º. Combine first five ingredients in a saucepan, stirring well. Cook over medium heat until syrup becomes clear and slightly thickened, stirring as needed to prevent sticking.

Pour into a 9-inch square baking pan coated with cooking spray.

In a separate bowl, combine margarine, sugar, flour and milk; blend well. Spoon topping over peaches.

Bake for 25 minutes or until golden brown.

Variation: You may use frozen peaches. To substitute for 2 cans of peaches plus juice, use 3 1/2 cups frozen unsweetened peaches, 1/2 cup water and 1/2 cup sugar.

Serving size: 1/3 cup
Analysis per serving: 189 Calories, 2 g Protein, 37 g Carbohydrate,
4 g Fat, tr Sat Fat, tr Cholesterol, 194 mg Sodium
Diabetic exchanges: 1 starch, 1 1/2 fruits & 1 fat

WALNUT AND SPICE CAKE

24 servings

Vegetable cooking spray
2 1/2	*cups all-purpose flour*
1 1/2	*cups granulated brown sugar*
1/2	*teaspoon salt*
1/4	*teaspoon ground mace*
1/2	*teaspoon ground cardamom*
1/2	*cup (1 stick) margarine, softened*
1/4	*cup chopped walnuts*
1	*teaspoon baking soda*
1	*egg*
1/4	*cup applesauce*
1	*cup nonfat buttermilk*

Glaze
1	*cup confectioners sugar*
2	*tablespoons skim milk*
1/4	*teaspoon vanilla extract*

Preheat oven to 350°. Coat 10-inch bundt pan with cooking spray. Stir together flour, sugar, salt, mace and cardamom in a large mixing bowl. Add margarine; mix until crumbly with pasty blender or fork.

Measure 1 1/2 cups of this dry crumb mixture into a small bowl; add walnuts and spread on bottom of the prepared bundt pan.

Stir together soda, egg, applesauce and buttermilk; mix well. Combine buttermilk mixture with remaining dry mixture. Pour this batter evenly over dry crumb mixture in bundt pan.

Bake for 40 to 45 minutes or until a wooden pick inserted in center comes out clean. ☺

Cool 10 minutes in pan; remove and let cool on a wire rack.

Transfer cake to a serving plate.

Combine glaze ingredients in a small bowl until smooth and drizzle over top.
Cut cake into 24 slices.

Serving size: 1 slice
Analysis per serving: 174 Calories, 2 g Protein, 31 g Carbohydrate,
5 g Fat, 1 g Sat Fat, 11 mg Cholesterol, 131 mg Sodium
Diabetic exchanges: 1 starch, 1 fruit & 1 fat

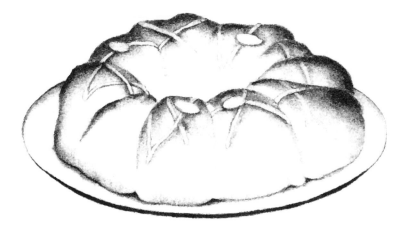

QUICK CHOCOLATE CAKE

24 servings

1/2	*cup (1 stick) margarine, softened*
1 1/2	*cups sugar*
1/2	*teaspoon baking soda*
2/3	*cup cocoa*
2	*cups self-rising flour*
2	*eggs*
1 1/2	*cups skim buttermilk*
1 1/2	*teaspoons vanilla extract*
Vegetable cooking spray	
1/4	*cup powdered sugar*

Preheat oven to 325°. Cream margarine and sugar in a large bowl, beating at medium speed with electric mixer until light and fluffy (about 5 minutes).

Add next 6 ingredients. Beat for 3 minutes.

Pour or spoon batter into a 13-x 9-x 2-inch baking pan coated with cooking spray. Bake for 35 to 40 minutes or until a wooden pick inserted in center comes out clean.

Cool completely in pan. When cool sprinkle with powdered sugar, and cut into 24 portions. Serve from pan if desired.

Serving size: 1 square
Analysis per serving: 140 Calories, 3 g Protein, 21 g Carbohydrate,
5 g Fat, 1 g Sat Fat, 22 mg Cholesterol, 190 mg Sodium
Diabetic exchanges: 1 starch, 1/2 fruit & 1 fat

OATMEAL APPLESAUCE COOKIES

This mixture can be spread in a shallow pan,
baked and cut into bars if desired.
4 1/2 dozen cookies

1 1/2	cups unsweetened applesauce
1	cup granulated brown sugar
1	egg
1	teaspoon vanilla extract
1/4	cup skim milk
1 1/2	cups all-purpose flour
1	teaspoon baking powder
1	teaspoon ground cinnamon
2	cups quick or old fashioned oatmeal
1	cup raisins

Vegetable cooking spray

Preheat oven to 350°. Combine all ingredients in a large bowl. Allow mixture to sit at least 15 minutes for oatmeal to soften. ☺

Drop the softened mixture by tablespoonfuls onto cookie sheets lightly coated with cooking spray. Bake for 10 minutes or until cookies are lightly browned on top.

Remove from pan and cool on a wire rack.

Serving size: 3 cookies
Analysis per serving: 125 Calories, 2 g Protein, 29 g Carbohydrate,
tr Fat, tr Sat Fat, 12 mg Cholesterol, 57 mg Sodium
Diabetic exchanges: 1 starch & 1 fruit

CHOCOLATE PIE

8 servings

Filling

1/3	cup cornstarch
1/3	cup cocoa
1	cup sugar
3	cups skim milk
2	eggs, separated
1	tablespoon margarine
1	teaspoon vanilla extract
1	6-ounce prepared graham cracker crust

Meringue

2	egg whites
1/2	teaspoon vanilla
1/4	cup sugar

Preheat oven to 425°. Place cornstarch, cocoa, and sugar in saucepan and stir to mix well. Gradually stir in milk. Cook over medium heat until very thick.

Remove from heat and mix 1 large spoonful of the hot pudding into the egg yolks which have been lightly beaten. Stir until blended.

Reduce heat to low. Slowly add egg yolk mixture to hot pudding, stirring constantly. Cook on low heat for 2 to 3 minutes while stirring. Remove from heat and stir in margarine and vanilla. Pour filling into crust. ☺

Beat egg whites in a small bowl at high speed of an electric mixer until soft peaks form. Add vanilla. Gradually add sugar and mix well. Spoon over pie and spread with a knife or spatula to cover.

Bake for 3 minutes or until lightly browned. Cool, then cut into 8 servings.

Serving size: 1 slice
Analysis per serving: 193 Calories, 4 g Protein, 31 g Carbohydrate,
7 g Fat, 3 g Sat Fat, 55 mg Cholesterol, 125 mg Sodium
Diabetic exchanges: 2 starches & 1 1/2 fats

Apricot-Topped
Fat-free Ice Cream

6 servings

1/3	*cup sugar*
3/4	*cup water*
1/2	*pound dried whole apricots (about 1 1/2 cups)*
1	*tablespoon lemon juice*
3	*cups vanilla fat-free ice cream*
1/4	*cup sliced almonds*

Bring sugar and water to a boil in a 1-quart saucepan. Add apricots, reduce heat and cook covered for 30 minutes or until apricots are tender.

Remove from heat and stir in lemon juice. Cool before spooning over fat-free ice cream. Top with almonds.

Serving size: 1/2 cup vanilla fat-free ice cream,
1/4 cup apricot topping and 2 teaspoons almonds
Analysis per serving: 222 Calories, 4 g Protein, 47 g Carbohydrate,
3 g Fat, tr Sat Fat, 0 mg Cholesterol, 41 mg Sodium
Diabetic exchanges: 2 starches, 1 fruit & 1/2 fat

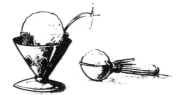

CHEWY DATE SQUARES

16 servings

4	*tablespoons margarine*
1	*cup granulated brown sugar*
3/4	*cup chopped dates*
2	*tablespoons chopped pecans*
1/2	*teaspoon vanilla extract*
1	*egg*
3/4	*cup self-rising flour*

Vegetable cooking spray

Preheat oven to 350°. Heat margarine in a 1-quart saucepan over medium heat just until melted.

Remove from heat. Stir in brown sugar, dates, pecans, vanilla and egg. Gradually add flour, stirring after each addition.

Spread batter in a 9-inch square baking pan coated with cooking spray. Bake for 25 minutes or until set and lightly browned.

Cool in pan before cutting into 16 squares.

Note: By gradually adding the flour last, you will find this easier to mix.

Serving size: 1 square
Analysis per serving: 128 Calories, 1 g Protein, 23 g Carbohydrate,
4 g Fat, 1 g Sat Fat, 16 mg Cholesterol, 98 mg Sodium
Diabetic exchanges: 1/2 starch, 1 fruit & 1 fat

CHOCOLATE CHIP PEANUT BUTTER BARS

16 servings

1/2	*cup sugar*
1/2	*cup granulated brown sugar*
4	*tablespoons margarine*
1/3	*cup chunky peanut butter*
1	*egg*
1/4	*cup skim milk*
1 1/2	*cups self-rising flour*
1/2	*cup mini chocolate chips*

Vegetable cooking spray

Preheat oven to 350°. Combine sugars, margarine, peanut butter, egg and skim milk in a medium bowl. Beat at medium speed with an electric mixer until creamy.

Add flour and mix well. Stir in chocolate chips. ☺

Spread batter in a 7 1/2 x 11 1/2 inch baking pan coated with cooking spray. Bake for 30 minutes or until lightly browned.

Cool in pan before cutting into 16 bars.

Serving size: 1 bar
Analysis per serving: 180 Calories, 3 g Protein, 25 g Carbohydrate,
7 g Fat, 2 g Sat Fat, 13 mg Cholesterol, 221 mg Sodium
Diabetic exchanges: 1 starch, 3/4 fruit & 1 1/2 fats

FROZEN STRAWBERRY CHIFFON DESSERT

9 squares

1	cup graham cracker crumbs
3/4	cup evaporated skim milk
1	10-ounce box frozen strawberries in light syrup, thawed
1/4	cup sugar

Spread graham cracker crumbs in a 9-inch square pan and set aside.

Chill evaporated skim milk several hours or overnight. Pour chilled milk into a large bowl; beat at high speed of an electric mixer until stiff. Add thawed strawberries and sugar; mix well.

Spoon or pour onto the graham cracker crumbs. Freeze.

Remove from the freezer about half an hour before serving to allow to soften before cutting into 9 portions. Serve immediately.

Serving size: 1 square
Analysis per serving: 105 Calories, 3 g Protein, 23 g Carbohydrate,
1 g Fat, tr Sat Fat, 1 mg Cholesterol, 89 mg Sodium
Diabetic exchanges: 1 starch & 1/2 fruit

HEAVENLY HASH

6 servings

1/3	cup fat-free sour cream
1	8-ounce can pineapple chunks, in its own juice, drained
2/3	cup chopped dates
1	cup mini-marshmallows
1	11-ounce can mandarin oranges, drained

Place the first 4 ingredients in a large bowl. Mix well.

Add mandarin oranges and stir very gently. Chill before serving.

Variation: In place of dates, you may use golden or regular raisins.

Serving size: 1/2 cup
Analysis per serving: 133 Calories, 2 g Protein, 33 g Carbohydrate,
tr Fat, tr Sat Fat, 0 mg Cholesterol, 14 mg Sodium
Diabetic exchanges: 1 starch & 1 fruit

STRAWBERRY SHORTCAKE WITH FAT-FREE ICE CREAM

16 servings

1/2	cup (1 stick) margarine, softened
1 1/4	cups sugar
2	eggs
1	teaspoon vanilla extract
2 1/4	cups self-rising flour
1	cup skim milk
	Vegetable cooking spray
1	quart vanilla fat-free ice cream
1	quart strawberries, washed, hulled, and cut into halves

Preheat oven to 325°. Cream margarine and sugar in a large bowl; beat at medium speed of an electric mixer until light and fluffy (about 5 minutes).

Add eggs and vanilla; beat 1 minute. Add flour and milk and beat for 2 minutes.

Pour batter into an 8 1/2- x 4 1/2 inch loafpan coated with cooking spray. Bake for 55 to 60 minutes or until a wooden pick inserted in center comes out clean. ☺

Remove from pan and let cool on a wire rack before cutting into 16 slices.

Just before serving, top each slice of cake with 1/4 cup vanilla fat-free ice cream and approximately 1/4 cup strawberries.

Any fruit can be used to top this cake.

Serving size: 1 slice
Analysis per serving: 248 Calories, 5 g Protein, 42 g Carbohydrate,
7 g Fat, 0 g Sat Fat, 33 mg Cholesterol, 288 mg Sodium
Diabetic exchanges: 1 3/4 starches, 1 fruit & 1 1/2 fats

APPLE CRISP

6 servings

Vegetable cooking spray
1   20-ounce can sliced apples, no sugar added
1/4   cup granulated brown sugar
1/4   cup all-purpose flour
1/4   cup oatmeal, quick cooking
1/4   teaspoon cinnamon
2   tablespoons margarine, melted

Preheat oven to 375°. Lightly coat an 8-inch square baking pan with cooking spray. Place apple slices in pan.

Mix remaining ingredients thoroughly. Sprinkle over apples. Bake 30 minutes or until topping is golden brown.

Serve warm and, if desired, with a topping of vanilla low-fat yogurt.

Serving size: 1/2 cup
Analysis per serving: 172 Calories, 1 g Protein, 34 g Carbohydrate,
4 g Fat, 1 g Sat Fat, 0 mg Cholesterol, 51 mg Sodium
Diabetic exchanges: 1/4 starch, 2 fruits & 1 fat

HONEY RICE AND FRUIT

8 servings

1	*cup cooked brown rice (cooked without salt or fat)*
1	*6-ounce package dried chopped mixed fruit*
1/2	*cup honey*
2	*tablespoons chopped pecans*
1	*cup fat-free sour cream*

Cook rice according to package directions without adding salt or margarine. Remove from heat.

Add fruit, honey, and pecans. Mix well. Cool for 1 hour at room temperature. ☺

Add sour cream and stir until well mixed. Chill before serving.

Serving size: 1/2 cup
Analysis per serving: 173 Calories, 3 g Protein, 38 g Carbohydrate,
1 g Fat, tr Sat Fat, 0 mg Cholesterol, 33 mg Sodium
Diabetic exchanges: 1 starch & 1 1/2 fruits

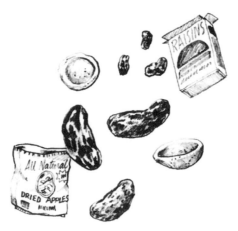

SPICY FRUIT BAKE

8 servings

1	*8-ounce can unsweetened apricot halves*
1	*16-ounce can unsweetened pear halves*
1	*15 1/4-ounce can unsweetened pineapple chunks*
3/4	*cup reserved juice from fruit*
1/4	*cup granulated brown sugar*
1/4	*teaspoon ground cinnamon*
1/4	*teaspoon ground nutmeg*
1	*tablespoon margarine, softened*
1/2	*cup low-fat vanilla yogurt*

Drain fruits, reserving 3/4 cup juice, and place fruit in a 2-quart casserole dish.

Combine reserved juice with brown sugar, cinnamon, nutmeg and margarine in a separate bowl. Pour juice mixture over fruit.

Bake at 350° for 20 minutes or until hot and bubbly.

Serve warm and top each serving with 1 tablespoon low-fat vanilla yogurt.

Serving size: 1/2 cup fruit mixture and 1 tablespoon yogurt
Analysis per serving: 128 Calories, 1 g Protein, 28 g Carbohydrate,
2 g Fat, tr Sat Fat, 1 mg Cholesterol, 29 mg Sodium
Diabetic exchanges: 2 fruits & 1/2 fat

LEMON CAKE PUDDING
(Pudding With Cake On Top)

6 servings

2	*eggs, separated*
1	*cup sugar, divided*
1/4	*cup lemon juice*
2	*tablespoons margarine, melted*
1 1/2	*cups skim milk*
1/2	*cup self-rising flour*
	Vegetable cooking spray

Preheat oven to 350°. Beat egg whites in a small bowl at high speed of an electric mixture until stiff; add 1/2 cup sugar; mix and set aside.

In a medium bowl mix the yolks, remaining sugar, lemon juice, margarine and milk. Add flour and beat until smooth. ☺

Combine egg white and egg yolk mixtures and mix on low speed just until blended.

Pour batter into a 2-quart baking dish coated with cooking spray. Bake for 45 minutes or until set. Do not over-brown.

Spoon into small bowls for serving.

Serving size: 1/2 cup
Analysis per serving: 247 Calories, 5 g Protein, 44 g Carbohydrate,
6 g Fat, 1 g Sat Fat, 72 mg Cholesterol, 204 mg Sodium
Diabetic exchanges: 2 starches, 1 fruit & 1 fat

MIXED FRUIT BREAD PUDDING

9 squares

6   *slices white bread*
Vegetable cooking spray
1/3   cup dried mixed fruit

1 1/2   cups skim milk
1/2   cup sugar
1   egg
1   egg white (reserve yolk for custard sauce)
1   teaspoon vanilla extract
1/4   teaspoon ground cinnamon

Preheat oven to 325°. Cut or tear bread into small pieces and place in an 8-inch square nonstick baking pan coated with cooking spray. Distribute dried fruit over bread cubes.

In a separate bowl, combine remaining ingredients and pour over bread and fruit. Let stand for 15 minutes.

Bake for 55 to 60 minutes or until puffed and set. Do not overbrown.

Cut into 9 squares. Serve warm with VANILLA CUSTARD SAUCE (page 211).

Serving size: 1 square with 2 tablespoons custard sauce
Analysis per serving: 167 Calories, 5 g Protein, 30 g Carbohydrate,
2 g Fat, tr Sat Fat, 29 mg Cholesterol, 137 mg Sodium
Diabetic exchanges: 2 starches & 1/2 fat

RAISIN BREAD PUDDING

9 servings

6   *slices raisin bread*
Vegetable cooking spray

1 1/2   *cups skim milk*
1/2   *cup sugar*
1   *egg*
1   *egg white*
1   *teaspoon vanilla extract*
1/4   *teaspoon ground cinnamon*

Preheat oven to 325°. Cut bread into 1-inch cubes and place in an 8-inch square nonstick baking pan coated with cooking spray.

Combine remaining ingredients in a separate bowl and pour over bread. Let stand for 15 minutes.

Bake for 55 to 60 minutes or until puffed and set. Do not over-brown.

Cut into 9 squares. Serve warm with VANILLA CUSTARD SAUCE (page 211).

Serving size: 1 portion pudding and 2 tablespoons custard sauce
Analysis per serving: 145 Calories, 4 g Protein, 28 Carbohydrate,
2 g Fat, tr Sat Fat, 29 mg Cholesterol, 117 mg Sodium
Diabetic exchanges: 1 starch, 1 fruit & 1/2 fat

Appendices

Contents

Appendix A
WHEN EATING IS DIFFICULT

If you are often unable to eat due to an illness or a condition which requires medications, you may find yourself struggling to get adequate amounts of the necessary nutrients. Older persons or people with chronic disease or arthritis may be taking numerous medications and must deal with a variety of symptoms which make it difficult to eat. Mouth sores, difficulty in swallowing, dulled taste and smell sensation, diarrhea and cramping, or just a lack of appetite can lead to a poor diet. Nausea, vomiting, constipation, heartburn, and fatigue can result in a less than adequate diet. Whatever the reason for not eating adequately, here are suggestions for making it easier.

Are You Just Not Hungry?

❑ Eat during the times you feel good. Eat a hearty breakfast and a substantial mid-morning snack. If you are really feeling good, prepare foods ahead to be eaten later when you might feel down. On good days, eat any time you are hungry, even if it isn't mealtime.

❑ Use foods that are easy to prepare. Canned, frozen, or convenience foods are often quick fixes. Choose foods that are easy to chew and digest. Follow the Dietary Guidelines in *Chapter 2* for healthful choices among convenience foods.

❑ Eat smaller, more frequent meals. You may become overwhelmed by a large plate of food. In between meals, snack on nutritious foods such as yogurt, cheese, muffins, peanut butter, raw vegetables or fruit.

❑ Don't drink liquids with meals. Coffee, tea and other non-caloric beverages can fill you up and prevent you from wanting to eat.

❑ Use nutritious liquids between meals. Juices, milk, milk-shakes and instant breakfast drinks can give you a nutrition boost. If you are lactose-intolerant, treat the milk with a lactase enzyme.

- ❑ Eat in a pleasant, relaxing atmosphere. Garnishes, attractive table settings, and an eating companion can make mealtime more enjoyable.

- ❑ Eat nutritious snacks. Keep low-fat cheese, peanut butter, canned fruits, and cereals handy for times when you feel like munching.

Is your mouth and throat dry?

- ❑ Be sure your physician and pharmacist are aware of all medications you are taking.

- ❑ Add moisture to the air with a vaporizer.

- ❑ Protect your lips with petroleum jelly.

- ❑ Stop smoking.

- ❑ Select food high in fluid content and drink beverages with dry foods.

- ❑ Artificial saliva is available. Discuss this option with your physician or registered dietitian.

- ❑ Chewing gum may be helpful.

Do You Feel Nauseated?

- ❑ Eat small meals. If you do eat less at mealtime, eat more frequently throughout the day.

- ❑ Avoid high-fat foods. Foods low in fat are easier to digest and leave the stomach faster than fatty, greasy foods.

- ❑ Choose salty foods over sweet ones, especially if you have nausea.

- ❑ Wear loose, comfortable clothes and get plenty of fresh air.

- ❑ Avoid activity right after eating.

Do You Have Chewing and Swallowing Problems?

❑ Eat softer foods that require little chewing and are easier to swallow like mashed potatoes, oatmeal, yogurt, scrambled eggs, cottage cheese, macaroni and cheese, and puddings.

❑ Use a blender to soften your favorite foods.

❑ Drink beverages and soups through a straw (except following tooth extraction).

❑ If your mouth or throat is sore, you may need to limit your use of spices, salt and acidic foods.

Feeling Too Tired To Eat?

❑ Choose convenient, easy-to-prepare food (see *Appendix B*). Rely on frozen dinners, canned biscuits, soups and vegetables, fat-free ice cream, cheeses, and sliced deli meats for quick fixes. Choose carefully to avoid too much fat and sodium, if you do this on a regular basis.

❑ Get some help, even just for one meal a day. Let friends, family, and organizations (such as Meals-On-Wheels) know your needs.

❑ Use time- and energy-saving appliances. Food processors, blenders, pressure cookers, microwave ovens and dishwashers save time in meal preparation and clean up which saves your energy for other activities.

❑ Eat and cook when you feel best. When you do cook, make enough for several meals and freeze it. It will be available for the times you don't feel like cooking. Many people have more energy in the morning and feel more like eating. If you do, take advantage and eat a hearty breakfast.

Is Diarrhea Causing You Trouble?

❑ Eat less fiber (roughage) in your diet during bouts of diarrhea. Cook fruits and vegetables instead of eating them raw. Stick with soft foods that won't further irritate the bowel. Avoid foods with seeds and tough skins, broccoli, corn, onions, and garlic.

❑ Foods like applesauce and bananas contain soluble fiber and may help reduce diarrhea.

❑ Avoid carbonated beverages, beer, beans, cabbage, broccoli, and other gas-producing foods. These can worsen cramps and bloating.

❑ Keep yourself hydrated by drinking plenty of water. But drink between meals rather than with meals. Drinking large amounts of juices and/or milk may worsen diarrhea. If you don't tolerate milk sugar (lactose), try milk with lactase enzyme added.

Is Constipation a Problem?

❑ Gradually increase the fiber in your diet. Add a variety of fruits and vegetables, whole grain breads and cereals, dried fruits (raisins, prunes or apricots), and nuts. If you can't chew or swallow these, chop them or put them into a blender.

❑ Try adding one or two tablespoons of bran to your foods. It often goes undetected in cooked cereals, casseroles and baked goods.

❑ Drink plenty of liquids. Eight to ten full glasses of water or other liquids without caffeine are needed each day. Prune juice and hot lemon water help some people (a squirt of lemon juice in 6-8 ounces of hot water).

❑ Set aside a specific time every day for trying to have a bowel movement.

❑ Incorporate light exercise, such as walking, into your daily regimen.

Is Heartburn a Problem?

❑ If you are a smoker, quit smoking.

❑ If you are overweight, lose weight.

❑ Don't eat within 2 to 3 hours before going to bed. Elevate the head of the bed 4 to 6 inches by using blocks or bricks.

❑ Avoid tight clothing and belts.

❑ Eat regular meals but reduce the size of the portions.

❑ Decrease fats, chocolate, alcohol, peppermint and spicy foods in your diet.

Are You Looking for Foods Which are Low in Fat?

If you have ongoing eating problems but don't need the extra fat in your diet, you will need to be more selective in your food choices.

Low-fat or nonfat yogurt, low-fat cottage cheese, 1% low-fat milk
Hot and cold cereals (except granola types)
Toast with jelly or honey (no butter)
Broth-based soups
Crab, white fish, shrimp, tuna packed in water
Spaghetti with meatless sauces
Veal, chicken, turkey breast and lean cuts of other meats - braised, roasted or cooked without added fat
Vegetables and vegetable juices
Fruits and fruit juices
Sauces, puddings or shakes made with skim milk
Angel food cake, Graham crackers
Popsicles, sherbet, nonfat frozen yogurt, sorbet
Fat-free, oil-free salad dressings, mayonnaise, and sour cream
Hard and jelly candies
Grated low-fat cheeses added to vegetables, casseroles, soups and sauces

If you are not sure why you have difficulty eating, discuss your eating problems with your physician. There could be a compounded medical problem. Making sure you get adequate nutrition during a prolonged illness or condition will improve your overall health.

Appendix B
CONVENIENCE FOODS

Getting a Balanced Meal

Convenience foods save time and energy in the kitchen. When carefully chosen, they can be incorporated as part of a balanced diet with a wide variety of foods.

Remember that when you use convenience foods, you have no control over the amount of fat or sodium that have been added. You do have control over mixes that call for added ingredients such as oils, milk, eggs or salt. You can simply omit salt, use low-fat milk, reduce oil or margarine by one fourth to one third or replace a whole egg with two egg whites.

Be sure to read the nutrient and ingredient labels. Reading nutrition labels can help you choose which foods are right for you. Thanks to revised labeling laws, most packaged foods have to provide standardized and accurate nutrition information. Refer to the example of a current food label on page 243.

The food label uses **Daily Values** (DVs). DVs serve as a basis for declaring on the label the percent of the Daily Value for each nutrient that a serving of the food provides. It also provides a basis for defining terms which can be used on a label, such as "high fiber." High fiber can be used if a serving of a food provides 20% or more of the Daily Value for fiber. The Daily Values (DVs) don't tell you what you should eat, they just give you an idea of how a product may or may not help you meet your nutritional needs. For most nutrients, except fat, you should try to obtain 100% of the DV.

The DVs are based on 2 components. One is **Daily Reference Values** (DRVs) and the other is **Reference Daily Intakes** (RDIs). The DRVs apply to fat, saturated fat, cholesterol, carbohydrate, protein, fiber, sodium and potassium. The RDIs are references based on the Recommended Dietary Allowances (RDAs) for essential vitamins and minerals.

DRVs are based on the number of calories an individual consumes in a day and only applies to adults. For the food label, 2,000 calories has been established as the number DRVs would be calculated. DRVs are based on the following:

> 30% of calories from fat (10% from saturated fat)
> 60% of calories from carbohydrates
> 10% of calories from protein
> Fiber based on 11.5 grams of fiber per 1,000 calories
> Cholesterol: 300 mg/day
> Sodium: 2,400 mg/day
> Potassium: 3,500 mg/day

The other nutrients that are shown on the label are limited to vitamins A and C, calcium and iron. The RDI for vitamin A is 5,000 international units (IU). The RDI for Vitamin C is 60 milligrams. Calcium's RDI is set at 1,000 milligrams, while iron is set at 18 milligrams.

To eliminate the confusion consumers might experience while looking at a label if it had both DRVs and RDIs, all of the values are referred to as a percent Daily Value (DV). The food label is designed to help you figure out how a food can fit into your diet.

Sample Food Label

Serving sizes are now more consistent across product lines, stated in both household and metric measures, and reflect the amounts people actually eat.

The list of nutrients covers those most important to the health of today's consumers, most of whom need to worry about getting too much of certain items (fat, for example), rather than too few vitamins or minerals, as in the past.

The label of larger packages must now tell the number of calories per gram of fat, carbohydrate, and protein.

Nutrition Facts

Serving Size ½ cup (114g)
Servings Per Container 4

Amount Per Serving

Calories 90   Calories from Fat 30

                     % Daily Value*

Total Fat 3g	**5%**
Saturated Fat 0g	**0%**
Cholesterol 0mg	**0%**
Sodium 300mg	**13%**
Total Carbohydrate 13g	**4%**
Dietary Fiber 3g	**12%**
Sugars 3g	
Protein 3g	

Vitamin A	80%	Vitamin C	60%
Calcium	4%	Iron	4%

* Percent Daily Values are based on a 2,000 calorie diet. Your daily values may be higher or lower depending on your calorie needs:

		Calories	2,000	2,500
Total Fat	Less than		65g	80g
Sat Fat	Less than		20g	25g
Cholesterol	Less than		300mg	300mg
Sodium	Less than		2,400mg	2,400mg
Total Carbohydrate			300g	375g
Fiber			25g	30g

Calories per gram:
Fat 9 • Carbohydrate 4 • Protein 4

New title signals that the label contains the newly required information.

Calories from fat are now shown on the label to help consumers meet dietary guidelines that recommend people get no more than 30 percent of their calories from fat.

% Daily Value shows how a food fits into the overall daily diet.

Daily Values are also something new. Some are maximums, as with fat (65 grams or less); others are minimums, as with carbohydrate (300 grams or more). The daily values for a 2,000- and 2,500-calorie diet must be listed on the label of larger packages. Individuals should adjust the values to fit their own calorie intake.

Understanding the Food Label

There are specific qualifications a product has to meet to use defined terms on the label. These terms can help you make better food selections.

FREE An amount that is "nutritionally insignificant" and can be labeled as zero.
CALORIE-FREE: fewer than 5 calories per serving
SUGAR-FREE: less than 0.5 grams per serving
SODIUM-FREE: less than 5 milligrams of sodium per serving
FAT-FREE: less than 0.5 grams of fat per serving, providing that it has no added ingredient that is fat or oil.
CHOLESTEROL-FREE: less than 2 milligrams of cholesterol per serving and 2 grams or less saturated fat per serving.
PERCENT FAT-FREE: refers to the actual fat-free weight of a food and may only describe foods that meet FDA's definition of low-fat or fat-free products. The higher the fat free percent the better choice the product is.

LOW Would allow frequent consumption of a food "low" in a nutrient without exceeding the dietary guidelines.
LOW-SODIUM: no more than 140 milligrams per serving
LOW-FAT: no more than 3 grams per serving
LOW-CALORIE: no more than 40 calories per serving
LOW IN SATURATED FAT: may be used to describe a food that contains 1 gram or less of saturated fat per serving.
LOW IN CHOLESTEROL: 20 milligrams or less per serving and the product can only have 2 grams or less of saturated fat per serving.

HIGH Is 20 percent or more of the Daily Value. A "Good Source" is 10% to 19% of the Daily Value.

MORE This term means that a serving of food, whether altered or not, contains a nutrient that is at least 10% of the Daily Value more than the reference food.

REDUCED This term means that a nutritionally-altered product contains 25 percent less of a nutrient or calories than the regular or reference product.
REDUCED-FAT: must contain at least 25 percent less of the fat of the reference food. For example, "Reduced fat, 25 percent less fat than our

regular brownie. Fat content has been reduced from 8 grams to 6 grams."
REDUCED-SATURATED FAT: must contain at least 25 percent less of the saturated fat of the reference food.
REDUCED-CHOLESTEROL: 25 percent less cholesterol per serving than its comparison food. The reduction in cholesterol must exceed 20 milligrams per serving. All claims of cholesterol content are prohibited when a food contains more than 2 grams of saturated fat per serving. The label of a food containing more than 11.5 grams of total fat per serving or per 100 grams of the food must disclose those levels immediately after any cholesterol claim.
REDUCED-SODIUM: The food must contain at least 25 percent less sodium than the regular product.

LESS   This term means that a food, whether altered or not, contains 25 percent less of a nutrient or calories than the reference food. For example, potato chips that have 25 percent less fat than regular potato chips could carry a "less" claim. "Fewer" is an acceptable synonym.

LITE/LIGHT   This descriptor can mean two things. First, that a nutritionally-altered product contains one-third fewer calories or half the fat of the reference food. If the food derives 50 percent or more of its calories from fat, the reduction must be 50 percent of the fat. Second, that the sodium content of a low-calorie, low- fat food has been reduced by 50 percent. In addition, "light in sodium" may be used on food in which the sodium content has been reduced by at least 50 percent. The term "light" still can be used to describe such properties as texture and color, as long as the label explains the intent; for example, "light brown sugar" and "light and fluffy".

FRESH   Can only be linked to raw food that has never been frozen or heated, or contains no preservatives.

LEAN AND EXTRA LEAN   Describes the fat content of meat, poultry, seafood, and game meats. Lean means less than 10 grams fat, 4.5 grams or less saturated fat, and less than 95 milligrams of cholesterol per serving. Extra lean means less than 5 grams fat, less than 2 grams saturated fat, and less than 95 milligrams of cholesterol per serving.

Frozen Foods

The frozen food section offers many choices; everything from plain frozen vegetables to complete gourmet meals. When choosing frozen food, remember that plain items are usually the lowest in calories, fat, sodium and price. Batters, breadings and deep-fat frying add fat and calories. Sauces and gravies can add additional sodium and fat. Low-fat and low-sodium varieties can be found and are made especially to fit into a healthful diet. Read labels to help you choose wisely.

Frozen dinners and entrees are some of the easiest and most convenient meals to use at home. All you need to add is a vegetable or salad, fruit, bread and a beverage. When your time and energy is limited, these products can offer a meal option without having to prepare meals from scratch. It is important to think about nutrition when choosing convenience foods, refer to Table 23 to identify those frozen dinners and entrees with no more than 12 grams of fat per serving. **Beware: Many of those listed are high in sodium.**

Frozen entrees and dinners can be high in sodium. Choose those with a lower sodium content. Remember, health advisory groups recommend that we limit our intake of sodium from 1,100 to 3,000 mg or less per day. Try not to exceed 1,000 mg per meal.

If you use a frozen dinner that is high in fat or sodium, balance it by using other low-fat and low-sodium foods during the rest of the day. It's the total daily diet that counts, not just one food.

Table 23: Low-fat Frozen Entrees, 12 grams of fat or less

Product: 1 serving	Calories	Fat (g)	Sat Fat (g)	% DV Fat %	Cholesterol (mg)	Sodium (mg)
Budget Gourmet: All Light & Healthy Entrees are low-fat.						
Healthy Choice:						
Chicken Enchilada Supreme	390	9	4	14	25	580
Chicken Fettuccine Alfredo	250	3	1	5	30	370
Chicken Picante	220	2	1.5	3	35	330

Table 23: Low-fat Frozen Entrees cont'd, 12 grams of fat or less

Product: 1 serving	Calories	Fat (g)	Sat Fat (g)	% DV Fat %	Cholesterol (mg)	Sodium (mg)
Country Glazed Chicken	200	1.5	.5	3	30	480
Country Herb Chicken	270	4	1.5	6	35	340
Sweet & Sour Chicken	310	5	1	8	50	250
Fettuccine Alfredo	240	5	2	8	10	430
Cheese French Bread Pizza	310	4	2	6	10	470
Pepperoni French Bread Pizza	360	9	4	14	25	580
Traditional Meat Balls	320	9	3	14	65	600
Traditional Swedish Meat Balls	320	8	4	13	35	460
Jennie-O:						
Chicken Breast Fillets	150	3.5	1.5	5	60	720
Extra Lean White Turkey Roast	120	3	1	5	55	780
Turkey Breast Fillet	120	1	0	1	45	680
Lean Cuisine (Stouffer's):						
Cheese Lasagna with Chicken Breast	290	8	2.5	13	40	560
Cheese Cannelloni	270	8	3.5	12	30	500
Cheddar Bake	220	6	2	10	29	560
Macaroni and Cheese	270	7	3.5	11	20	550
Baked Chicken	250	6	.5	9	30	590
Chicken Italiano	270	6	1.5	9	40	560
Honey Mustard Chicken	250	4.5	1	7	50	460

Table 23: Low-fat Frozen Entrees cont'd, 12 grams of fat or less

Product: 1 serving	Calories	Fat (g)	Sat Fat (g)	% DV Fat %	Cholesterol (mg)	Sodium (mg)
Chicken						
Fettuccine	290	8	3.5	12	40	570
Mandarin						
Chicken	270	6	1	9	30	520
Fettuccine						
Primavera	260	8	2.5	12	15	580
Lasagna	290	8	4	11	35	560
Rigatoni	180	4	1.5	6	20	560
Oriental Beef	250	8	3	12	30	480
Swedish						
Meatballs	290	8	3	13	55	590
Lean Pockets:						
Chicken Fajita	260	8	3	12	40	770
Glazed Chicken						
Supreme	240	7	2.5	11	30	600
Turkey, Broccoli						
& Cheese	260	8	3	12	35	710
Turkey, Ham						
& Cheddar	260	7	3	11	35	810
Smart Cuisine:						
Chicken and						
Vegetable	190	1	0	1	20	1020
Chicken Fettuccine						
Alfredo	270	6.5	2	9	20	820
Chicken Divan	260	8	2	12	25	870
Imperial Chicken	230	0	0	0	15	930
Pasta in Wine						
& Mushroom Sauce						
with Chicken	290	7	2	11	30	670
Beef w/ Peppers	210	3.5	1.5	5	15	1140
Beef Stroganoff	290	7	4	11	35	580
Jumbo Stuffed						
Shells	200	2	1	3	10	380
Swanson:						
Grilled Chicken in						
Garlic Sauce	270	7	3	11	30	640

Table 23: Low-fat Frozen Entrees cont'd, 12 grams of fat or less

Product: 1 serving	Calories	Fat (g)	Sat Fat (g)	% DV Fat %	Cholesterol (mg)	Sodium (mg)
Tombstone:						
Light Vegetarian Pizza	240	7	2.5	11	10	500
Tyson:						
Chicken Picatta	190	3	1	5	50	530
Honey Roasted Chicken	190	3	.5	5	45	460
Van De Kamp's:						
Crisp & Healthy Fish Sticks	180	3	.5	4	25	440
Weight Watcher's: All Smart Ones entrees are 99% fat-free.						
Broccoli & Cheese Baked Potato	250	7	2	11	10	590
Cheese Manicotti	260	7	3.5	11	30	570
Italian Cheese Lasagna	300	8	3.5	12	30	550
Macaroni and Cheese	260	6	2	9	20	550
Barbecued Glazed Chicken	190	3.5	1	5	20	340
Stuffed Turkey Breast	240	8	3	12	20	590
Fettuccine Alfredo with Broccoli	220	6	2.5	9	15	540
Tuna Noodle Casserole	240	7	2.5	11	15	580
Penne Pasta	290	9	2.5	14	15	550
Lasagna	270	7	3	11	35	570
Macaroni & Beef	230	5	1.5	8	15	540
Spaghetti and Meatballs	290	6	1.5	9	15	560
Deluxe Combo Pizza	380	11	3.5	17	40	550
Pepperoni Pizza	390	12	4	18	45	650

Canned and Packaged Foods

❑ Canned and packaged foods are easy to store, have a long shelf life and can shorten meal preparation time. Many may be high in sodium, fat or sugar. Here are some guidelines to keep in mind to make your selections healthly ones. Refer to Table 24 for low-fat canned and boxed entrees.

❑ Canned vegetables are higher in sodium than fresh or frozen plain vegetables. When using canned vegetables, choose no-salt-added ones. Such products are found throughout the canned goods aisles.

❑ Canned and dry soups are usually high in sodium and creamed ones are high in fat and sodium. 99% fat-free soups are lower in sodium and are very useful when making casseroles. Read labels and compare to make good choices.

❑ For more fiber, choose soups made with beans or peas. Incorporating small amounts of leftover vegetables is not only thrifty but provides a nutritional boost.

❑ Dry and box mixes for entrees, side dishes and sauces prepared according to package instructions are often high in fat and sodium. Prepare them without adding margarine, oil or salt. Use only half of the seasoning packet to reduce sodium.

❑ Use reduced-calorie, fat-free and reduced-sodium varieties of mayonnaise, salad dressings and spreads. Brands vary; select one that is tasty to you.

❑ Choose water-packed tuna over tuna packed in oil to lower fat and calories.

❑ Choose canned fruits packed in juice or water rather than in syrup to reduce sugar and calories.

❑ Choose unsweetened fruit juices. Many juice drinks or punches contain little fruit juice and use sugar as the main ingredient.

Table 24: Low-fat Boxed and Packaged Entrees
12 grams of fat or less (be aware that sodium is very high)

Product: 1 serving	Calories	Fat (g)	Sat Fat (g)	% DV-Fat (%)	Cholesterol (mg)	Sodium (mg)
BOXED MIXES						
Dinner Sensations (Betty Crocker):						
Sweet & Sour Chicken	330	4	1	6	35	320
Top Shelf (Hormel):						
Beef Ravioli	300	9	4	14	45	800
Glazed Chicken Breast	200	5	1.5	8	50	910
CANNED ENTREES						
Chef Boy Ar Dee:						
Cheese Tortellini	230	1	0	2	15	770
Meat Tortellini	260	3	1	.5	50	810
Beef Ravioli	230	5	2.5	8	20	1150
Mini Beef Ravioli	230	5	2	8	20	1120
Beefaroni	260	7	3	11	25	1070
Chun King:						
Chicken Chow Mein	100	3	1	5	15	1080
Hot & Spicy Chicken	110	2.5	.5	4	15	880
Beef Chow Mein	110	2.5	1	.04	15	920
Hot & Spicy Beef	110	2.5	1	.04	15	1020
Dinty Moore:						
Turkey Stew	150	3	1	5	25	1080
Franco American:						
Beef Raviolios	300	10	4	15	25	1160
Spaghettios	190	2	.5	3	5	990
Spaghetti in Tomato Sauce with Chesse	210	2	1	3	5	1020

Table 24: Low-fat Boxed and Packaged Entrees, cont'd
3 gm fat/100 gm (Be aware that sodium is very high)

Product: 1 serving	Calories	Fat (g)	Sat Fat (g)	% DV-Fat (%)	Cholesterol (mg)	Sodium (mg)
Hormel:						
Turkey Chili with Beans	200	3	1	5	50	1170
Vegetarian Chili with Beans	200	0	0	0	0	830
LaChoy:						
Beef Chow Mein	110	1.5	1	2	10	760
Beef Pepper Oriental	100	2.5	.5	4	10	970

Cereals and Breads

Breakfast cereals are a regular item on many shopping lists. Here are some tips to help you make healthy choices:

❑ Cereals give information about their fiber, sodium and sugar content. Comparing labels can help you choose one that is low in added sugar and sodium, and high in fiber.

❑ Choose a cereal that provides 5 grams of dietary fiber in the size serving which you normally eat. This choice will put you well on your way to reaching the daily 25-35 grams of fiber recommended by health advisors.

❑ Granola cereals may be high in calories, fat and sugar. Look for reduced-fat or fat-free granola cereals.

❑ Regular and quick-cooking hot cereals are lower in sodium than instant cereals, especially if you omit salt during cooking. Adding fruit such as figs, dates or raisins to oatmeal and other whole-grain cereals will also add fiber.

❑ Whole-grain breads have more fiber, but deciding which bread to choose can be difficult. Look for whole-grain flour such as whole wheat or rye as the first ingredient on the label.

Cookies, Chips and Snacks

Bakeries in supermarkets now include bread products and sweet baked goods that vary in fat, sugar and and fiber content. Healthful choices may be available. Ask questions and read labels; refer to Table 25 for healthful crackers and snacks.

❑ Baked goods such as cakes, cookies, brownies, pastries, croissants, buttery rolls and biscuits provide more fat and sugar than plain breads, bagels or English muffins.

❑ Look for snack foods that do not contain animal fats such as lard or beef tallow. These fats, as well as palm, palm kernel or coconut oils, are high in saturated fat. Generally crackers that feel greasy are higher in fat than others.

❑ Choose unsalted crackers, pretzels, nuts, seeds, and chips to reduce sodium intake.

Table 25: Low-fat Snack Foods

Product: 1 serving	Calories	Fat (g)	Sat Fat (g)	%DV-Fat (%)	Cholesterol (mg)	Sodium (mg)
CHIPS						
Louise's Fat-free Potato Chips:						
Barbecue Chips	110	0	0	0	0	180
Maui Onion	110	0	0	0	0	180
Original	110	0	0	0	0	180
Vinegar & Salt	100	0	0	0	0	300
Nabisco:						
Mr. Phipp's Fat-Free Pretzel Chips	100	0	0	0	0	630
Mr. Phipp's Original Pretzel Chips	120	2.5	0	4	0	630

Table 25: Low-fat Snack Foods, cont'd

Product: 1 serving	Calories	Fat (g)	Sat Fat (g)	%DV-Fat (%)	Cholesterol (mg)	Sodium (mg)
Mister Salty, Fat-Free	110	0	0	0	0	400
Keebler:						
Munch 'ems Salsa Chips	140	4	1	6	0	260
Munch 'ems Chili Cheese Chips	140	4	1	6	0	430
Munch 'ems Sour Cream & Onion	130	3	.5	.55	0	390
COOKIES						
Nabisco:						
Fat-free Fig Newtons	100	0	0	0	0	115
Fat-free Apple Newtons	100	0	0	0	0	60
Fat-free Cranberry Newtons	100	0	0	0	0	90
Fat-free Strawberry Newtons	100	0	0	0	0	90
Rippin' Good: All Smart Bake flavors are fat-free.						
Smart Bake Devil's Food Cookies	100	0	0	0	0	170
Keebler:						
Animal Crackers	190	5	2	0	8	110
Vanilla Wafers Reduced-Fat	130	3.5	.55	0	0	140
Elfin Delights	70	0	0	0	0	80
Snack Well's (Nabisco):						
Truffles	60	0	0	0	0	60
Double Fudge Cookie Cakes	50	0	0	0	0	70
Cinnamon Graham Snacks	110	0	0	0	0	90

Table 25: Low-fat Snack Foods, cont'd

Product: 1 serving	Calories	Fat (g)	Sat Fat (g)	%DV-Fat (%)	Cholesterol (mg)	Sodium (mg)
Chocolate Chip Cookies	130	3.5	1.5	5	0	170
Chocolate Sandwich Cookies/Creme	130	2.5	.5	0	0	220
Regular Creme Sandwiches	110	2.5	.5	4	0	100
CRACKERS						
Nabisco:						
Ritz Crackers, Reduced-fat	70	2.5	.5	4	0	135
Ritz with Whole Wheat	70	2.5	0	4	0	120
Wheat Thins, Reduced-fat	120	4	.5	6	0	220
Triscuit, Reduced-fat	130	3	.5	4	0	180
Harvest Crisps, Italian Herb	130	3	.5	.55	0	460
Harvest Crisps, 5-Grain	130	3.5	.5	6	0	300
Snack Well's (Nabisco):						
Wheat Crackers	60	0	0	0	0	170
French Onion	120	2	0	3	0	290
Zesty Cheese	120	2	.5	3	3	350
Cracked Pepper	60	0	0	0	0	150
Classic Golden Crackers	60	1	0	1	0	140
Cracker Jack:						
Fat-free Butter Toffee Caramel Corn	110	0	0	0	0	95
Fat-free Original Caramel Corn	110	0	0	0	0	85
Louise's Fat-free Caramel Corn						
	100	0	0	0	0	80

❑ The following crackers (any brand) are low in fat:

Graham crackers
Rye crisps
Soda/Saltine crackers
Melba toast
Oyster crackers
Rice cakes
Zwiebach toast

❑ Other low-fat snacks include fat-free pretzels, plain popcorn, frozen yogurt, fruit ice, fudge bars such as Fudgesicles®, pops such as Popsicles®, fat-free ice cream and sherbet.

Carryout Foods

If you are willing to pay for convenience, items from the deli or restaurants can be served as the main part of a meal, with added fruit and vegetables or a salad. Select your takeout foods carefully. Go easy on fried foods and high-sodium sauces, such as soy sauce or dipping sauces. For information on ingredients of takeout items prepared at the supermarket, ask the counter manager.

❑ Salad bars have expanded and many include foods like soups and chili. These foods vary widely in how they are prepared and in the nutrients they provide. Ask questions.

❑ Pizza may include vegetable, bread, dairy and meat components which can contribute to a well-balanced meal. Choose low-fat toppings such as part-skim Mozzarella, Canadian bacon and lots of vegetables to reduce fat content. Skip the extra cheese.

It is up to you to determine whether or not you should use a convenience item. The time and energy you have for food preparation, cost of the item, nutritional contributions and its taste are all factors you will have to consider. You know your time and energy constraints better than anyone else and must decide what best meets your needs.

Resource List

The following organizations and companies offer free nutritional information and may be of help to you.

* **American Dietetic Association Center for Nutrition & Dietetics.**
#1-800-366-1655. Call Monday-Friday, 8 am to 8 pm (CT). Features timely recorded nutrition messages and the opportunity to speak directly with a Registered Dietitian.

* **Betty Crocker Baking Hotline.**
#1-800-328-6787 or 1-800-328-1144. Monday-Friday, 7:30 am to 5:30 pm (CT). Staff members respond to nutrition, baking, storage, recipe and General Mills product questions.

* **Butterball Turkey Talk-Line.**
#1-800-323-4848 Monday-Friday, 8 am to 6 pm (CT.) Features recorded messages on turkey preparation and the opportunity to talk with a home economist.

* **Land O'Lakes Holiday Bakeline.**
#1-800-782-9606 November 1 to December 24 only! (includes weekends and holidays) 8 am to 6 pm (CT). Features home economists ready to answer your holiday baking and cooking questions. Callers can also receive a free holiday leaflet.

* **Pillsbury Consumer Relations.**
#1-800-767-4466 Monday-Friday, 8 am to 6 pm (CT). Staff members respond to nutrition, baking, storage, recipe and Pillsbury product questions.

* **Seafood Hotline.**
#1-800-328-3474 Monday-Friday, 9 am to 5 pm (ET) Staff will respond to questions on purchasing, preparation, storage and nutritional value of seafood products.

* **USDA Meat and Poultry Hotline**
#1-800-535-4555 Monday-Friday, 9 am to 5 pm (ET) Features timely recorded food safety information and the opportunity to speak directly with a home economist or dietitian.

References

* AN INTRODUCTION TO THE NEW FOOD LABEL, USDA-FSIS
41, DHHS Publications, No. (FDA) 94-2271, October 1993.
* FOCUS ON FOOD LABELING, FDA Consumer, May 1993.
* SHOPPING FOR FOOD AND MAKING MEALS IN MINUTES
USING THE DIETARY GUIDELINES, USDA, Home and Garden
Bulletin No. 232-10, 1990.
* THE NEW FOOD LABEL FDA BACKGROUNDER, December 1992.

INDEX

Reorder Form

NEW! THE ESSENTIAL ARTHRITIS COOKBOOK: Kitchen Basics for People with Arthritis, Fibromyalgia and Other Chronic Pain and Fatigue. Excellent nutrition information, medication tables, photos and illustrations, overcoming energy-robbers, when eating is difficult, useful resources and tools, 120 low-fat recipes that save time and energy! 288 pages, Hardcover with Double-wire O binding.
$24.95 each..*Send me*____*for a total of $*_____

NEW! HEALTHY MEXICAN COOKING: Authentic Low-Fat Recipes. Delicious, traditional Mexican foods with few ingredients, practical preparations and moderate to low calories. Plus, glossary, special mail-order section and more than 160 wonderful, authentic recipes! 256 pages, Softcover with Ota-binding.
$14.95 each..*Send me*____*for a total of $*_____

Also from Appletree Press Inc.
COOKING ALA HEART The Classic! With more than 80,000 copies in print, its recipes are always hailed as original, delicious and easy to make. Selected by the editors of the Harvard Medical School health letters, this book features two chapters of sound nutrition information and over 400 recipes! Softcover, 456 pages.
$19.95 each..*Send me*____*for a total of $*_____

WHAT'S FOR BREAKFAST? The easiest way to stop cheating yourself of a good breakfast! Over 100 delicious and easy recipes divided by preparation time: Super Quick, Quick and Worth the Effort — all low in fat and calories. The "Pro-Carb" Connection to hold off hunger, special shopping sections and menus for all occasions!
$13.95 each..*Send me*____*for a total of $*_____

SHIPPING
Add $4.00 for one book, $5.00/2 books, $6.00/3 books, $7.00/4-6 books.......*total $*_____

Minnesota residents...Add 6.5% tax $_____

TOTAL ENCLOSED $_____

Circle one: Check   Visa   MasterCard

Card #_____Exp. Date_____

Ship to: _____

Street address_____

City, State and Zip Code_____

Mail your order to:
Appletree Press Inc.   Suite 125   151 Good Counsel Drive   Mankato, MN 56001
or Order Toll Free #800-322-5679